Men'sHealth

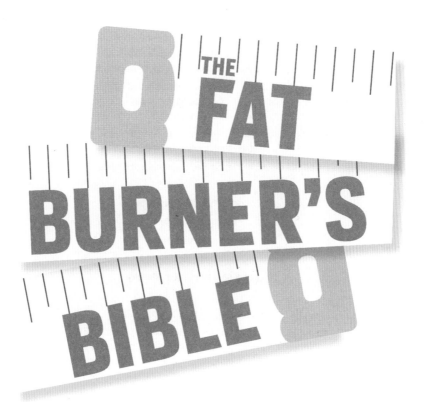

THE FAT BURNER'S BIBLE

This book is intended as a reference volume only, not as a medical manual. The information given here is designed to help you make informed decisions about your health. It is not intended as a substitute for any treatment that may have been prescribed by your doctor. If you suspect that you have a medical problem, we urge you to seek medical help.

The information in this book is meant to supplement, not replace, proper exercise training. All forms of exercise pose some inherent risks. The editors and publisher advise readers to take full responsibility for their safety and know their limits. Before practising the exercises in this book, be sure that your equipment is well-maintained and do not take risks beyond your level of experience, aptitude, training and fitness. The exercise and dietary programmes in this book are not intended as a substitute for any exercise routine or diet that may have been prescribed by your doctor. As with all exercise and dietary programmes, you should get your doctor's approval before beginning.

Mention of specific companies, organisations, or authorities in this book does not imply endorsement by the author or publisher, nor does mention of specific companies, organisations, or authorities imply that they endorse this book, its author, or the publisher.

Internet addresses and telephone numbers given in this book were accurate at the time it went to press.

Men's Health is a registered trademark of Rodale Inc

Editor-in-Chief **Morgan Ress**

Editor **Tom Stone**

Art Editor **Paul Aarons**

Production **Roger Bilsland**

Editorial Assistant **Clem Murphy**

For photography credits see page 254

Hearst-Rodale, 33 Broadwick Street, London, W1F 0DQ

Printed in the United Kingdom

To reorder a copy of this book visit menshealth.co.uk/books
or call 0844 848 1601

For a digital version download the Men's Health UK app from the Apple Newsstand and go to 'special editions'

ISBN 978-0-9568190-6-0

HEARST - *Rodale* | **UK**

Dedicated to all the fat burners
who have told their stories in the
pages of *Men's Health* and
inspired others to lose weight

CONTENTS

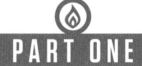

PART ONE

GETTING STARTED

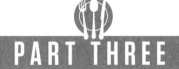

PART FOUR

MAINTENANCE

CASE STUDIES

Throughout this book you'll find inspirational stories from men who fought fat so successfully they appeared in the pages of *Men's Health*. Here's where to turn to get their first-hand accounts...

EXTRAS

FOREWORD

LET'S SAY YOU RUN INTO an old friend whom you haven't seen in a while. He has lost three stone, looks about 10 years younger, and is bursting with the kind of energy that you wouldn't mind having. Wouldn't you be just a little bit curious to know how he did it?

We would. And that's how this book came about. You see, for the past 10 years in almost every issue of *Men's Health* magazine we've published a simple success story like that about one man's struggle to lose weight and shape up. They appear on our Fat Burner of The Month page where we chronicle his transformation from fat man to fit man.

In recent months this page has grown into its own section – The Fat Burner's Bible (or FBB for short). It is one of the most-read parts of the magazine, but there's been so much to say that we can't always fit it all in. What's more, single case studies and new research don't give a full picture. It's often useful to reference older stories and principles to get a better idea of the best ways to burn fat, particularly if you're new to the concept. That's why we thought it was high time we published a definitive weight-loss book, compiling everything we've learned, and our readers have taught us, over the years.

What this book does is make things simple. If you want the best information on how to burn fat, this is where to come. Instead of having to trawl the web, filtering fact from fiction, or searching through your dog-eared back issues of *Men's Health* to work out the most effective ways to shed pounds, you just need this book. How can we be so confident? Because all the information in here is based, not only on science, but on real men with busy lives who've proved these techniques work. In this book we'll be revisiting the stories of our most successful and inspirational fat burners. But, of course, in picking our favourites we also looked at the successes of dozens of other men who graced our pages since 2002 and reviewed yet more case histories from menshealth.co.uk. What we noticed was a pattern. Our big belly losers all used the same handful of techniques to drop three, four, sometimes even 15 stone!

The Fat Burner's Bible is based on those tips and techniques and the groundbreaking science that supports them. And it is your best tool for finally winning your battle with weight and taking off that belly of yours for good. This plan isn't about a special food or counting calories or fancy fitness gadgets. It's about real men doing old-school exercise at home. It's about eating really good food – food that tastes great, fills you up and satisfies your hunger so you won't overeat. What's more the myriad get-back-in-shape solutions we've included take into account your ever-changing goals and circumstances – so you'll always have new ways to get your best body ever and keep it for life.

Most importantly, if you are overweight, *The Fat Burner's Bible* will help you to significantly improve your health and lower your risk of developing diabetes or suffering from heart disease. That's why we are so proud of this *Men's Health* book and believe it is so important. The latest NHS figures show obesity kills more than 30,000 people in the UK every year, with your help we can reduce that figure, and this book is a step towards making that happen.

PART
ONE

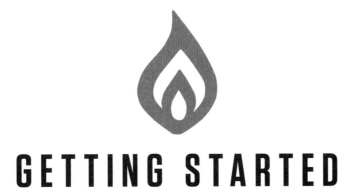

GETTING STARTED

①
THE
SECRETS
OF SUCCESS

THE JOURNEY TO AN LEANER, HEALTHIER BODY STARTS HERE

YOU MAY HAVE BOUGHT THIS BOOK because you are feeling a bit flabbier than a few years ago and you want to get back in shape. Or perhaps you have struggled with your weight for years and you are concerned about your health. Whatever your personal weight and fitness situation *The Fat Burner's Bible* will help you. That's a promise. We've seen it work for others. For nearly 20 years *Men's Health* has researched and published the very latest weight-loss science. The advice from the magazine has been used time and time again by readers to burn fat fast. This book brings together the very best tips we've ever published, and to prove they really do work, introduces the real men who have used them to transform their bodies.

OFTEN WE DON'T NOTICE WE'RE PUTTING ON WEIGHT. It happens gradually. There's no sudden change when we look in the mirror in the morning. Our jeans might get a bit tighter, but as soon as we've bought a new pair we forget about it. It's all too easy to put the extra pounds down to advancing years – an inevitable consequence of getting older that's impossible to do anything about. But that simply isn't the case. Too much fat isn't natural, it's extremely unhealthy. That means that ultimately, if you do nothing about it, it could kill you.

Sometimes we need a wake-up call before we take action. Often that might be something dramatic like someone we know dying too young. Tragic events like this tend to make you focus on what should really always be on top of your mind – things like your family, your purpose in life and your health. You start thinking: I'm not invincible. That could happen to me. It is high time I started taking better care of myself.

Most of us should. Today, 60% of Brits are overweight and nearly a quarter are classified as obese. It's no secret that being overweight can dramatically increase your risk of diabetes, high blood pressure, heart disease, gallbladder disease, sleep aponea and cancer. But it may surprise you to learn that new research, published in the journal *Health Affairs*, has established that being obese is a greater threat to your health than smoking or living in poverty. Researchers studying more than 111,000 heart attack patients found that while the average age of a first heart attack was 74.6 years in the leanest patients, it was 58.7 years in the obese.

"The leading theory in cardiology right now is that the fat tissue is actually producing factors that precipitate heart attacks," says study author Dr Peter McCullough, a cardiologist and chief of nutrition and prevention medicine at William Beaumont Hospital in Michigan. Dr McCullough says that a person with a Body Mass Index of more than 40 can expect a heart attack 12 years earlier than a person with a Body Mass Index (BMI) of 25 to 30. (For an explanation of BMI, see opposite.)

Once you've got the motivation to lose weight, you're already half way to achieving your goals. That's not to say it's going to be easy. Changing eating habits that you've acquired over many years

MEASURE YOURSELF

TWO EASY SELF-TESTS TO HELP YOU BEAT FAT

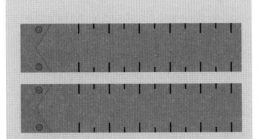

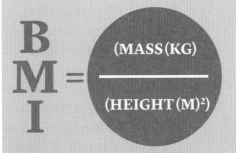

$$BMI = \frac{(MASS\,(KG)}{(HEIGHT\,(M)^2)}$$

Take the Tape Test for your most reliable measure of weight loss

Wrap a measuring tape around your abdomen so that the bottom of it touches the tops of your hips. Standing in front of a mirror will help you make sure the tape is positioned correctly, parallel with the floor. Don't suck in – let it all hang out. Stand straight and exhale as you pull the tape taut against the skin (without compressing it). A waist size of 40 inches or over for men and 35 inches or over for women is considered high risk for type 2 diabetes, heart disease, stroke and cancer.

Calculate your Body Mass Index for a rough check on your fat levels

This is a way of roughly calculating your body fat based on your height and weight. The formula for working it out is above, but it's often easier is to use a free online calculator. Type "BMI Calculator" into your search engine or try this one: tinyurl.com /nhsbmicalculator. A BMI of 30 or greater indicates obesity, 25 to 29.9 means overweight, and 18.5 to 24.9 is normal weight. One major limitation of this measurement is that if you are muscular, you'll have a high BMI even though you are not actually overweight.

is never going to be. That said, with the help of *The Fat Burner's Bible* it is possible to make a difference to your body in just one week (see Chapter Four for how it can be done). And once you've done that your sore body will start to feel pretty good. Some of the quickest successes will come in the beginning of a disciplined workout/diet regime, so use them to further stoke your motivation and keep you going in the weeks and months to come. You'll soon be running faster, sleeping better and feeling more energized and happy than you have done for years.

Real-World Results

If you are still finding it difficult to picture how the new you will look, take inspiration from the accomplishments of the men in this book. They will inspire you any time your motivation is flagging. *The Fat Burner's Bible* is based on the real-world examples of these readers whose stories have been chronicled in *Men's Health* in the past. They are living proof that the tips we are publishing here really work. We've also packed in as much of the latest weight-loss science from the world's best researchers, so when you begin your fat-burning regime you can be confident it's not only tried-and-tested but also ratified by experts.

Draw inspiration from men like Mike Hare of Cambridgeshire who at nearly 28 stone could hardly get out of the house, let alone walk to the shops. A serious car accident woke him up to the fragility of life and he embarked on a fitness programme that saw him lose over half his bodyweight – an incredible 15 stone. Now he's a keen marathon runner and describes his life as "infinitely better."

Or consider Dave Leather, who lost nearly seven stone to become a *Men's Health* Cover Model Competition finalist. His university diet of pizza and beer made him grow to 21 stone, but after going to the gym and getting serious about his nutrition, he discovered a new way of life and is loving every minute of it.

Then there's Adam Hall from Croydon, who fooled himself into thinking he was fit because he played a bit of American football. When his 44in waist sidelined him from the game he knew it was time to take action. He lost 10in off his waist in a year.

This book is filled with examples of people like these, who share their weight-loss strategies and personal tips from their journey to better health. Our case studies are real stories, of real people, who chose to shed their excess weight and start a healthier and more confident way of life.

GYM TIP

Don't exercise alone. Train with friends and you'll lose a third more weight than if you go to the gym alone, according to researchers at the University of Pennsylvania.

The Six Secrets of Weight Loss

How did so many men and women lose so many pounds? We were curious to know exactly how, too, so we reread every Fat Burner of the Month story going back 10 years, searching for the common strategies that have helped all of these men and women lose weight. Not only were we once again inspired by their stories, but we discovered something surprising: we noticed the same six weight-loss techniques over and over again. Here they are. Adopt all of them and you're bound to drop a few pounds very quickly:

1 — **96 percent** cut right back on foods with refined flour and added sugars, like those found in juices, fizzy drinks, white bread, rice, biscuits and cakes, substituting more fruits, vegetables, and fibre-rich whole grains.

2 — **93 percent** ate more lean protein and healthy fats.

3 — **90 percent** did muscle-building resistance exercises three or more times a week.

4 — **88 percent** did cardio exercises like running, cycling, and swimming, or regularly played sport.

5 — **85 percent** found that portion control is a crucial part of their weight-loss strategy.

6 — **75 percent** ate more often – four to six times a day – spacing their calories out to keep their metabolisms high.

What we also discovered about the above techniques, when we delved even deeper, is that every one of these real-world strategies is backed by the latest research on exercise, nutrition and weight loss. They work in the lab and they work at home. We've built this book around these principles. Turn the page for the full lowdown on how we've designed the most-effective weight-loss programme

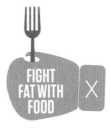

FIGHT FAT WITH FOOD

Drink grapefruit juice. You'll lose up to 4lb (2kg) in 12 weeks, thanks to its insulin-lowering enzymes, says the California Department of Nutrition and Metabolic Research.

YOUR ULTIMATE FAT-BURNING PLAN

YOU KNOW THIS BOOK IS BASED ON SCIENCE, and you know *Men's Health* readers prove it works every month. Here's how it will work for you. We've turned all that experience into a three point plan to guarantee you'll lose weight fast. Familiarise yourself with the basic principles here, then you'll be ready to embark on the body-changing plan. The programme consists of...

 The Seven-Day Quick-Start You're ready for action, but to ramp up your motivation even further this plan delivers results very fast.

 The Workouts Weight loss is accelerated by resistance work. But gyms put some people off. That's why we've developed a bodyweight regime you can do at home.

 Real Meals No matter how hard you exercise you won't lose weight unless you eat properly. So we've made easy recipes for every occasion.

The Seven-Day Quick-Start

 Starting on page 73 you'll find this day-by-day schedule of how to eat and exercise. We'll tell you exactly what to do. No thinking. Just follow the plan and you'll feel it working in just seven days.

You'll start each day with the Two-Minute Drill – eight quick moves designed to spark your metabolism. Then you'll eat a satisfying breakfast. Do these two things and you'll set yourself up for all-day fat burning. There's even a shopping list for the week. By the weekend you'll be establishing patterns of healthy habits that will soon become a natural part of your life.

The Fat-Burning Workouts

Part Two of this book has a complete set of fat-burning workouts you can do without a gym membership. They are centered around the Bodyweight 100 – a simple circuit of exercises you can do them anywhere. No gear needed. Each rep is designed to boost metabolism and build muscle in the least amount of time possible. It'll add several pounds of lean muscle to your frame in a few weeks. And that's important not only because you'll look great but also because one pound of muscle requires 50 calories per day just to maintain itself on your skeleton, even when it's not engaged in anything physical. Add just 2lb (1kg) of muscle and you'll burn 100 more calories per day even before you exercise.

As you progress through this section you'll be given the option of stepping up the pace by repeating this workout, or even getting down the gym or investing in some weights. But you can always return to the Bodyweight 100. It is a cornerstone of this programme and superbly effective at shifting flab.

And, of course, no fat-burning regime would be complete without some cardio. In this book you'll find the best ways to make your running, cycling or swimming as efficient as possible.

How To Make Your Own Real Meals

These recipes in Part Three are what make *The Fat Burner's Bible* different from other diets whose underlying theme is sacrifice and abstinence. We take favourite foods – steak, pizza, chilli, burgers, even burritos – and develop delicious recipes to satisfy your taste buds while also sticking to the principles of good nutrition. So you'll fill up without filling out.

Best of all, each Real Meal will provide you with the right mix of protein (to build muscle and burn calories), fat – yes, tasty fat (to keep you satisfied for a long period of time with fewer cravings!) – and fibre to keep you burning fat and prevent your body from storing it right where you don't want it – your belly.

GYM TIP

Play squash for an hour. You'll burn 1,035 calories – which is more than you would playing any other sport.

HOW TO KEEP YOUR EYES ON THE PRIZE

IT IS OUR SINCERE HOPE that this book will provide you with motivation you need to revamp your diet, start exercising in the correct way, improve your overall health and ultimately burn a lot of excess fat. And that you'll make those six strategies on page 19 a central part of your new lifestyle. But it all starts with desire and commitment. If you've bought this book and read this far you probably already have a desire to change your body. But maintaining that desire can be tricky. So here are some simple ways to ensure you won't give up. Do these now, and you will boost your chances of success dramatically...

FIND A PHOTOGRAPH OF YOU AT YOUR HEAVIEST and stick it somewhere you'll see it often. It'll serve as a reminder to put down those crisps and go for a run. Many readers who've ended up with their success stories printed in the pages of *Men's Health* say they found the 'fat photo' strategy one of the most effective forms of motivation.

NEXT, STEP ON THE SCALES and write your current weight on today's date on a calendar. You'll weigh yourself at the same time of day, and record the result every day. Why? Because a study at the Weight Control and Diabetes Research Center in Providence, Rhode Island, found that people who weighed themselves every day at the same time of day were 82 percent more likely to keep their weight off than people who didn't use scales. Positive feedback encourages positive action.

FINALLY, MAKE THE PROMISE on the opposite page to yourself. Sign it and date it. It might seem silly seeing as you're probably the only person who's going to see it. But studies show that people who sign a pledge are more likely to follow through with commitments. Once you've actually put your name to something, it's more likely to stick. It's about accountability.

FAT
BURNER'S
BIBLE

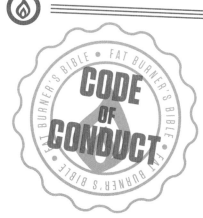

CODE OF CONDUCT

I promise to . . .

1. Eat a protein-rich breakfast daily to spark my metabolism and fill me up.

2. Follow the Bodyweight 100 exercise and intervals programme and start my day with the Two-Minute Drill.

3. Eat four to six small meals and snacks every single day.

4. Replace processed carbohydrates with wholegrains and reduce all complex carbs after 6pm. And to eat more fruit, vegetables, protein and a little fat.

5. Refrain from drinking alcohol for the next four weeks.

SIGNED ....

DATE ....

CASE STUDY

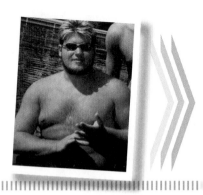

Dave Leather struggled with his weight, then he learnt a thing or two about nutrition and got a *Men's Health* cover-model body

"JUNK FOOD STALLED MY FAT BURNING"

Dave Leather's story is one of the most inspiring ever published in *Men's Health*. Not only did was he a Fat Burner of the Month, he also went on to be a finalist in the Cover Model Competition. A double whammy that has never been repeated. "I didn't even realise I was getting fat – it happened over 10 years," says Dave. "I was chubby as a child, but not fat. Then I went to university, ate pizzas and drank a lot – I got bigger than ever."

As he watched his weight increase Dave battled with it in vain, but he now realises that one of the major reasons for

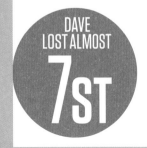

DAVE LOST ALMOST

7ST

has lack of success was that he didn't have a proper grasp of nutrition. "I'd cut down on food," he says. "But I failed because I didn't know the difference between fats, proteins, carbs and sugars." Turn to Chapter Eight for some of the latest science on fat-burning superfoods.

BOXING CLEVER

With the nutritional side of his weight loss regime failing to get off the ground, Dave managed to start losing weight with exercise – without even meaning to. "I got a job at a supermarket and lost weight by accident. I was shifting heavy boxes until 10pm. The only problem was that I was too tired to cook after that so I was still eating junk. I only lost 7lbs (3kg) in six months, but the important thing was that I realised I could lose weight."

Burning fat can be hard work. That's why it's important to take motivation from every small victory and not to let anything slow you down. That's what Dave did.

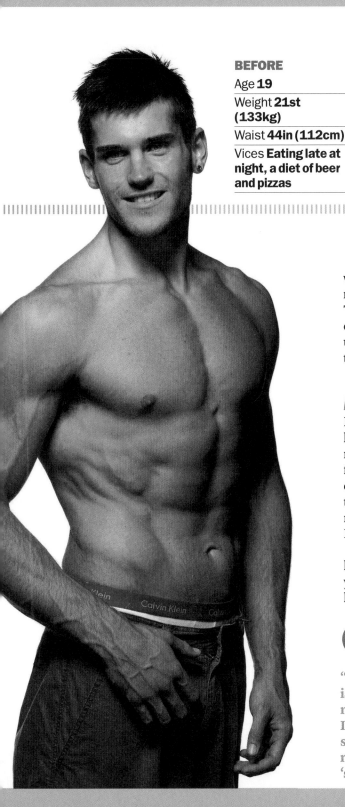

BEFORE		AFTER
Age **19**		Age **21**
Weight **21st (133kg)**		Weight **14st 4lb (90kg)**
Waist **44in (112cm)**		Waist **33in (84cm)**
Vices **Eating late at night, a diet of beer and pizzas**		Victories ***Men's Health*** **cover-model competition finalist**

"A year later I'd lost six stone, which gave me even more motivation to keep going further. That summer I spent every day of the six-week break from university in the gym. I needed to tone up: I loved the results."

A NEW BODY

During Dave's summer of weight lifting he got serious about his nutrition. "I now avoid saturated fat and try to eat 30-50g protein every three hours when I'm training hard, and five small meals a day when I'm not. Also, I set myself realistic goals."

Doing one virtuous thing will lead to other good habits. So if you go to the gym you're more likely to eat healthy food.

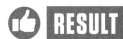 **RESULT**

"Losing weight and getting fit is more than physical: it's my new way of life. I love the gym. I run 6.5km twice a week, and swap workouts regularly – muscles need to constantly be 'surprised' to grow."

② AVOID THE EVERYDAY FAT TRAPS

> ## KNOWING WHAT PUT THE WEIGHT ON CAN HELP YOU TAKE IT OFF

YOU REALLY CAN'T FATHOM HOW MUCH YOU CAN EAT in a single day unless you keep track with pencil and paper. Give it a try. There's a blank food diary at the end of this chapter, which will help you to do just that. We guarantee this exercise will be an eye-opener.

Not only will it be illuminating, it's proven to help you to lose weight. A study in the *American Journal of Preventive Medicine* found the simple act of keeping a food diary can double a person's weight loss. Scientists asked subjects to record what they ate and then monitored their weight. "The more food records people kept, the more weight they lost," says lead researcher Dr Jack Hollis. This chapter will help you to spot the worst offenders in your food diary: the products and habits that are destroying our waistlines.

AT SOME POINT WE'VE ALL PROBABLY LOOKED IN THE MIRROR at our ample abdomens and thought, 'Oops! I look like I swallowed a small child! I ought to do something about that!' What we're critiquing in that mirror is how heavy we look. Maybe you have a date coming up. Or you're trying on a new suit. Or a beach holiday is around the corner and you want a David Beckham six-pack instead of that pie-crumb catcher.

How we look is important to our self-esteem, to our careers, to our love lives. But, there is a more important reason to be concerned with losing that gut. It's simply not healthy. Here's why.

The average man – that's you – is home to about 30 billion fat cells. Think of them as extremely tiny water balloons. But instead of being filled with water, they are filled with oily fats (lipids). Our bodies produce these fats, and we also get them from food.

Your fat cells are designed to be a reservoir for energy when you need it. But, if you get more fat than you need for energy, those cells expand like balloons and can divide. You can shrink fat cells but you can't get rid of them, which is why losing weight can be so tough. Unfortunately, in men unwanted fat tends to collect in our abdomen creating an apple- or pear-shaped body.

Give your gut a poke right now. Does it jiggle? Is it soft like pudding or could you bounce a cricket ball off of it? (we're assuming you're not the owner of a rock-hard six-pack). Soft and protruding or hard and protruding. Those are the two basic types of male potbellies, and one is much worse to have than the other. The soft kind is made up of subcutaneous fat, meaning it's located just under the skin in front of the abdominal muscles. Nobody likes this fat. You want it to vanish. Still, it's not as bad to have as the other kind.

The round and hard type of belly is made up of visceral fat, which forms around your internal organs. Fat that's hard up against your most crucial body parts is not a good thing. It secretes harmful compounds that raise blood pressure, spike blood sugar, and lead to inflamed arteries. All you have to know is that the bigger and harder your belly, the larger your visceral fat cells and the more active they are at secreting these harmful substances.

A protruding belly of 40 inches or more is one of the markers of a condition known as metabolic syndrome or prediabetes. The

NEW WEIGHT-LOSS SCIENCE

THE ONE-WORD SECRET TO FAT BURNING

Say "I don't eat pies" rather than "I can't eat pies" and you'll be eight times more likely to resist them. Scientists at the Universities of Houston and Boston proved this by trying to tempt 120 subjects with food over a 10-day period. The study authors explain that saying "I don't…" gave participants 'ownership' of the idea, where as "I can't…" suggested something beyond the subject's control was responsible for their actions. When we feel empowered we're more likely to stick with an idea.

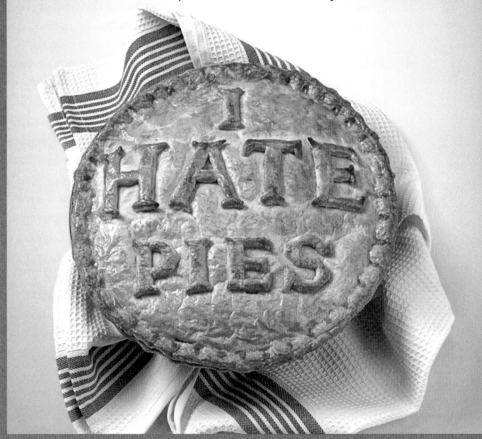

PSYCHOLOGY

other signs are high blood pressure, high triglycerides (fat in your blood), high blood sugar, and low HDL (good) cholesterol. Having a big belly and any two other markers means you have metabolic syndrome and should see your doctor.

According to Diabetes UK, 7 million people in Britain are living with prediabetes. It's a condition associated with every major age-related illness, including erectile dysfunction, Alzheimer's, blindness, kidney failure, cancer and heart disease. Untreated, prediabetes can turn into full-blown type 2 diabetes. In fact, having this condition increases your chances of developing diabetes fivefold and doubles your risk of a heart attack.

What exactly is diabetes? Basically, it's your body's inability to process sugar properly. But to fully understand this disease, it helps to know how the body uses food for energy.

When your body digests food, it turns carbs into glucose: the fuel that powers your cells. But glucose can't get into your body's cells on its own. It needs help from insulin, a hormone secreted by your pancreas. Insulin opens the door to certain cells and moves sugar from the blood into your organs. It is also insulin's job to deal with the fats we get from foods like meat, dairy products and vegetable oils. Insulin transports these fatty acids from the bloodstream into the body's tissues, where they are either used for energy or stored.

The pancreas is an unsung hero of all this, and it deserves our praise. But the way we eat often confuses this highly efficient organ. Here's how: let's say you pop out of the office at lunch for a chicken and mayo sandwich, crisps and cola, and then maybe you have a slice of chocolate cake because it's Linda from accounts' 30th birthday and you want to be a 'team player.' Suddenly, your system has much more energy than it can use right away, so insulin moves in to help. It hauls that surplus glucose into your liver, where it's turned into glycogen, and it takes the fatty acids from the blood to your fat cells, where they're saved as triglycerides (blood fats).

This flood of insulin drives your blood sugar lower, which makes you feel hungry again. For what? More carbs. Some biscuits, perhaps, or a chocolate bar. The cravings are similar to those a drug

EASY LIFESTYLE TWEAK

Take lunch breaks away from your desk. You'll consume 250 fewer calories in a day than if you eat and work, according to a recent study in the *American Journal of Clinical Nutrition*.

NEW WEIGHT-LOSS SCIENCE

HOW TO USE EVERYDAY ITEMS TO JUDGE PORTIONS

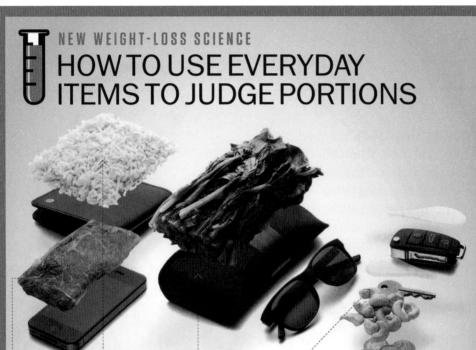

Dial up your protein portion

"A slab of beef the size of an iPhone is ideal for a balanced meal," says nutritionist Mayur Ranchordas. Meat is rich in leucine, an amino acid that jolts your metabolism. At 110 calories, you can almost burn off a portion this size with a quick game of Farmville.

Cash in on complex carbs

"Wholemeal pasta, fresh egg noodles and basmati rice provide plenty of energy in a form that won't spike your blood sugar," says Ranchordas. A lunchtime serving of cooked rice about the size of your wallet will chalk up a healthy 200 calories.

Keep an eye on green veg

Your portion should be about the size of your sunglasses on their case. "Cover half your plate with low-calorie vegetables," says dietitian Lyndel Costain. That's a mere 25 calories: a weight-loss prospect so bright, you may need to put those shades back on.

Find the key to dressing well

Swap sugary sauces for olive oil. "A drizzle of extra-virgin, about the size of two keys, will provide you with an ample amount of monounsaturated fat," says Costain. It's a fuss-free dressing that's proven to lower your cholesterol.

Pocket your omega-3 dose

"When it comes to fat, go nuts," says Ranchordas. "Walnuts, Brazils and cashews all have a slow digestion rates, so they'll increase your feelings of satiety." Serve up an amount equivalent to a handful of coins – just don't confuse the two.

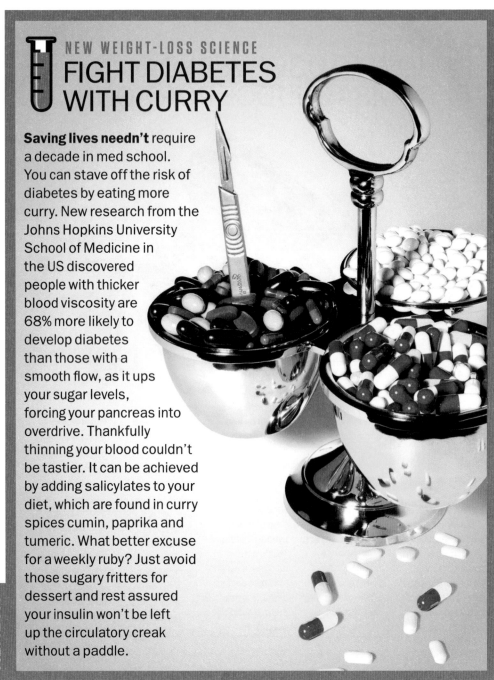

NEW WEIGHT-LOSS SCIENCE
FIGHT DIABETES WITH CURRY

Saving lives needn't require a decade in med school. You can stave off the risk of diabetes by eating more curry. New research from the Johns Hopkins University School of Medicine in the US discovered people with thicker blood viscosity are 68% more likely to develop diabetes than those with a smooth flow, as it ups your sugar levels, forcing your pancreas into overdrive. Thankfully thinning your blood couldn't be tastier. It can be achieved by adding salicylates to your diet, which are found in curry spices cumin, paprika and tumeric. What better excuse for a weekly ruby? Just avoid those sugary fritters for dessert and rest assured your insulin won't be left up the circulatory creak without a paddle.

addict experiences. And the process continues. Blood sugar jacks up from the new carbs, the pancreas dutifully responds with more insulin, and so on. Over time, this recurrence can lead to insulin resistance. You need more and more insulin to do the same job.

Type 2 diabetes cases have rocketed globally because of the way we eat. Eventually, the insulin manufactured by the pancreas becomes ineffective – that's diabetes. Once you have diabetes, you have to closely monitor your blood sugar levels and manage blood sugar with oral insulin or injections. If blood sugar isn't managed effectively, you can lose 5-10 years of your life and put yourself at great risk for blindness, nerve damage, amputation, impotence, kidney disease, stroke, and heart disease. Now you know why you should appreciate your pancreas.

Belly fat is also a major risk factor for cancer. A study in the *New England Journal of Medicine* concluded that virtually all forms of cancer are more prevalent in overweight people, and 15 percent of all cancer deaths could be tied to being overweight. What's fat got to do with cancer? Simple answer: it upsets the body's natural hormonal balance, making tissue an easier host for tumours.

As if that weren't enough, an unchecked fat belly automatically builds an even fatter belly by changing the very core of what makes you a man – testosterone. That's the male hormone tied to red blood cell production, muscle development and sexual functioning. A 20-year study tracking 584 men published recently in the *Journal of Clinical Endocrinology and Metabolism* found that a 4-point increase in Body Mass Index (BMI) accelerates your natural decline in testosterone by 10 years. This dip in the male hormone corresponded to an average gain of 2st 2lb (13.5kg) for a man of average height.

Know what that feels like? Grab a 12.5kg dumbbell and walk around for 10 minutes. Pretty tough. Well, that's a kilogram short of the extra work that you're asking your heart to do 24/7 when you are that much over your ideal weight. See page 17 for more on BMI and how to measure it, along with tips on how to measure your belly and reliably track your weight loss progress.

EASY LIFESTYLE TWEAK

Never sleep in a warm room. Turning down the thermostat not only means you'll sleep more soundly, you'll body will burn more fat to keep warm, too. Optimum bedroom temperature at night is 17°C.

JUST HOW DID BRITAIN GET SO FAT?

We could fill this entire chapter with the dangers of visceral fat and obesity, but you get the (bleak) picture. Instead, let's learn how we as a nation let ourselves go. That knowledge will help you to avoid the fat traps that you may be falling into and show you how to get rid of your gut and live a healthier and longer life. Here are our Top 5 reasons for the UK's growing weight problem:

1. We Eat The Wrong Food, Too Quickly

We Brits are officially the fattest people in Europe, according to a Department of Health survey, with a quarter of us classed as obese. Even the average British man has a BMI of 29 (5ft 9in tall, but weighing 12st 9lb), which means he is just one point off falling into the 'obese' range and is most definitely overweight. While many other nations in Europe aren't exactly saints on the nutrition front (Germans love sausages and the Italians eat tonnes of pasta) they all differ from us Brits in that they tend to have a slower, more considered approach to mealtimes. A recent survey commissioned by rural insurance firm Cornish Mutual found that over half of UK families no longer eat together at least once a day. What this means is that we think less about both the quality and quantity of our meals, and just grab whatever we fancy. So we end up eating big portions of processed, fat filled or deep fried food. Our European cousins have more sensibly sized portions and are more likely to have fresh fruit and veg on the side.

Are you part of that national trend? A simple at-home exercise will paint a clear picture of both how much you eat and exactly what you're putting in your mouth. We refer you once again to the food diary pages at the end of this chapter (page 48-49). Keep it for as long as you can. Even one day will reveal a lot about what you are putting in your body. Remember that study on the effectiveness of food diaries we told you about at the beginning of the chapter? That was one of the largest and longest-running weight-loss

NEW WEIGHT-LOSS SCIENCE
CHANGE YOUR PLATE TO EAT LESS

Buy a few coloured dishes and you'll eat 200 fewer calories per meal – which means 2lb (1kg) of weight loss over a month. Researchers at Georgia Institute of Technology in the US found that if you serve food on a plate with contrasting colour (eg mashed potato on a blue plate) you dish up 10 percent less than you would if using a similarly coloured plate. What's more, the effect is accentuated if you match your plate colour to your tablecloth. The researchers cited the cause of this phenomenon as the Delboeuf illusion, which says that our perception of the size of an object is affected by what it's placed on or near to. It could tip the weight-loss scales in your favour.

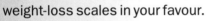

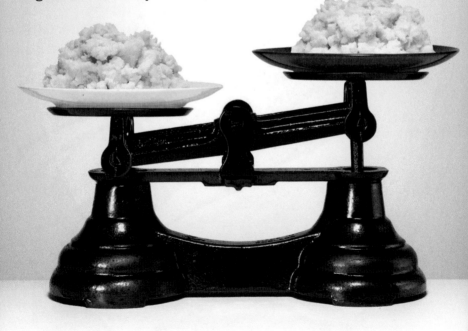

PSYCHOLOGY

RUN AWAY FROM HUNGER

Exercising to lose weight may not be the most revolutionary notion, but here lies a new rationale for championing Asics over Atkins. Aside from liquefying calories, Brazilian scientists at the University of Campinas have observed that exercise heightens the activity of the neurons that control feelings of fullness; ensuring you eat slowly and steadily. A 30-minute pre-work jog may leave you coveting breakfast, but will keep your hands out of the office biscuit tin later on.

maintenance surveys ever conducted. Doctors at the Kaiser Permanente Center for Health Research in Portland, Oregon, compared the different approaches to maintaining weight loss of 1,685 overweight or obese adults over 20 months, and found that people who kept track of their meals lost twice as much weight as those who didn't.

So start filling in your food diary today. It could be one of the most powerful weapons in your fight against fat. You don't have to use the pages in this book, you can scribble it on a napkin, write it on a calendar or input it into your smartphone. Just make sure you do it, one way or another. "It's the process of reflecting on what we eat that helps us to become aware of our habits and hopefully change our behaviours," says Dr Keith Bachman, a researcher at Kaiser Permanente's Weight Management Initiative

2. Our Portions Are Enormous

Have you been to an Italian restaurant lately? Just think about what you see on your plate after you've already had basket of garlic bread and maybe even a starter. Your waiter finally brings the main course. A huge doughy pizza, sometimes with extra cheese stuffed into the crust... and then there's the tiramisu. This could be one meal easily in excess of your guideline daily 2,500 calories – if you eat it all (thanks to Mum and Dad, who grew up during the post-war years and taught us to clean our plates). But they shouldn't feel guilty for laying guilt on us. Blame the savvy marketers who created the enormous portions and the extra-value meals.

Thanks to the big plates we're getting when we eat out, we've build a culture of 'more is better' where 'supersize me' is our mantra when we order. And this has confused our sense of a proper serving size. Studies show that when people are asked to describe how much they eat, they invariably underestimate. Then there is the buffet phenomenon. When we are faced with an abundance of food and food choices, we tend to serve ourselves more than we need. One Rutgers University study measured the amount of food people served themselves from a breakfast buffet. Then they

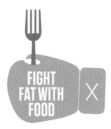

FIGHT FAT WITH FOOD

Eat 'good' fats to burn fat. Eggs and beef from grass-fed cows contain high levels of the fat conjugated linoleic acid (CLA). A study published in the *International Journal of Obesity* found increasing CLA intake reduces belly fat.

compared the results to a similar study conducted 19 years earlier. The recent study participants served themselves 16 percent more toast with jam, 43 percent more orange juice, 28 percent more milk for their cereal, and 19 percent more cornflakes than the similar group did nearly two decades earlier.

Even diet experts who should know better mess up portion sizes. In a recent Cornell University study, nutritionists who were asked to serve themselves ice cream at a party using large bowls and spoons dished out about 31 percent more than those who were given smaller bowls and spoons.

3. Added Sugars Lurk Everywhere

Not only are we eating more food, but we are eating more carbohydrates such as processed grains, potatoes, corn and sugar. A recent study by the Medical Research Council and the University of Cambridge found that we dramatically underestimate the amount of sugar we eat each day. Some Britons were eating as much as 207g – 52 more spoonfuls than the Guideline Daily Amount. The problem is that it's not just chocolate and cakes that contain a lot of sugar, it's often hidden in seemingly 'healthy' food like juice, bread, condiments, frozen dinners and cereals. And it's not just raw sugar we're eating more of. It's also the highly refined flour found in white bread, pasta, and breakfast cereals. Unlike protein, fat, and fibre – which have little if any impact on blood sugar – these refined carbohydrates quickly break down in our bodies and cause a fast increase in our blood-sugar levels, which in turn causes an insulin spike. Ultimately a bowl of white pasta quickly becomes a bowl of sugar once it's inside your body. But you can fight back with a little knowledge about Glycaemic Index and Load.

Glycaemic Index (GI) rates foods based on how quickly the body turns their carbohydrates into sugar (or glucose to be precise) and absorbs it into the blood. Glucose, the purest form of sugar, has the highest GI of 100. Your body has to very little work to do in order to break it down, so it gets into your bloodstream extremely quickly.

Focus on the specifics of your workout (ie how to do each exercise) rather than your reasons for doing it (ie burning fat). A study in the *Journal of Applied Biobehavioral Research* found that this will lead to more effective weight loss.

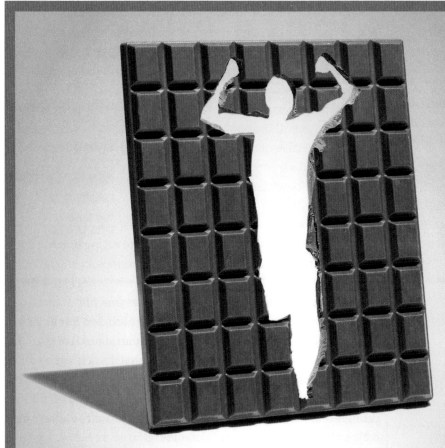

NEW WEIGHT-LOSS SCIENCE
EAT MORE CHOCOLATE TO LOSE MORE POUNDS

If you're trying to shrink your gut, you might think buying small, individually wrapped chocolates such as Celebrations would be a smart move. But new research shows you'll actually eat more with these tiny treats because their mini-measure size fools us into forgetting about portion control. Next time you want to treat yourself, it's best to opt for a whole bar of your favourite instead. Not a kilo slab of Dairy Milk, mind.

HIDDEN SUGARS

Sugar isn't always easy to spot. If you see any of these on an ingredients list, read 'sugar'

GLUCOSE

SUCROSE

MALTOSE

DEXTROSE

HONEY

GLUCOSE/FRUCTOSE SYRUP

FRUIT CONCENTRATE

NATURAL CANE

Be especially wary of these foods, which often hide the white stuff

YOGHURT

JELLY

TINNED FRUIT

PASTA SAUCE

SOUPS

SAUSAGES

SALAD DRESSINGS

PEANUT BUTTER

CRACKERS

FROZEN DESSERTS

Low GI foods are complex carbohydrates that your body takes longer to break down and they are therefore absorbed less quickly. Low GI foods include carrots (GI of 39) and porridge (GI of 55). Anything with a GI of 55 or below is considered 'low'. It's generally better to get most of your carbs from low GI sources as it means you get a slow release of energy that is easier to use up. If you get all your glucose at once the chances are your body won't be able to use it all, so it will store whatever is left over as fat.

But GI doesn't tell the whole story. While it's an excellent way of gauging how quickly your body absorbs carbohydrate, it doesn't actually tell you how much a typical portion contains. To do that you need to use Glycaemic Load (GL), which rates foods on a scale of 1-60 based on their GI alongside total carbohydrate content in an average portion. Watermelon for example has a high GI due to its natural sugars, however it has a very low GL of 4 because one slice contains very little in the way of carbs and is mostly water. High GL foods have a rating of 20 or more; low GL foods a rating of 10 or less.

So, next time you're shopping, look out for low GI or GL foods and also be aware that sugar can lurk in the most unexpected places. See the chart above for some common hiding places.

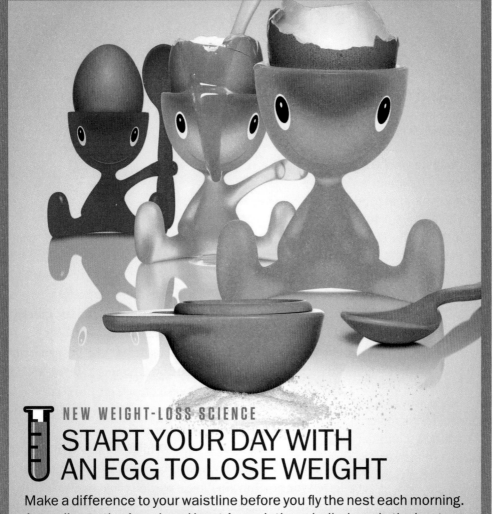

START YOUR DAY WITH AN EGG TO LOSE WEIGHT

Make a difference to your waistline before you fly the nest each morning. According to the American Heart Association a boiled egg is the best way to start your day. It will provide the ideal combination of increased fullness and prolonged energy release, so you'll be less likely to opt for a sugary snack, mid-morning. The AHA has also removed its previous limits on weekly egg consumption as long as you watch your dietary cholesterol from other sources. In fact, the average egg contains only 1.5g of fat, and 72.5% of what you're tucking into is pure protein. Cracking stuff!

NUTRITION

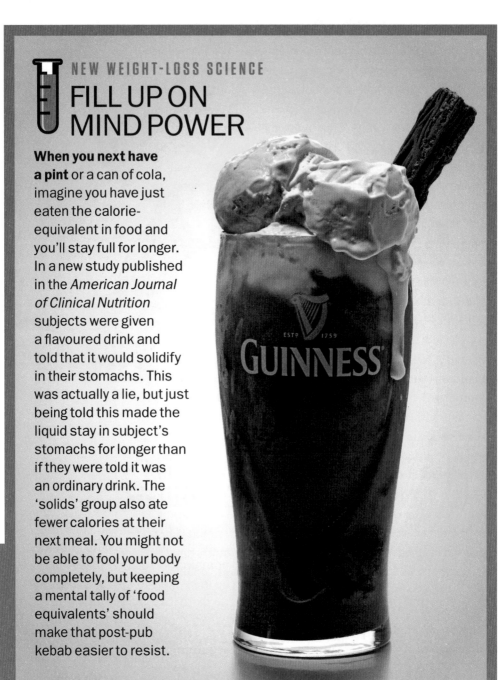

NEW WEIGHT-LOSS SCIENCE
FILL UP ON MIND POWER

When you next have a pint or a can of cola, imagine you have just eaten the calorie-equivalent in food and you'll stay full for longer. In a new study published in the *American Journal of Clinical Nutrition* subjects were given a flavoured drink and told that it would solidify in their stomachs. This was actually a lie, but just being told this made the liquid stay in subject's stomachs for longer than if they were told it was an ordinary drink. The 'solids' group also ate fewer calories at their next meal. You might not be able to fool your body completely, but keeping a mental tally of 'food equivalents' should make that post-pub kebab easier to resist.

4. We Drink Our Calories

It's easy to forget about the calorie content of drinks. Particularly when we're down the pub having a good time with our mates. But it's worth remembering that alcohol is hugely calorific. According to the NHS the average wine drinker in England takes on around 2,000 calories from alcohol every month. Five pints of lager a week adds up to 44,200 calories a year. That's the same as eating 221 doughnuts. Drinks are especially stealthy in this calorie war because the brain interprets liquids as less filling than solid food. When Purdue University in the US gave subjects foods in both liquid and solid forms, people consumed far more calories when they ate food in liquid form than when they ate solid food. However, you can turn this brain/body anomaly around, and use it to help you lose weight. See the latest science, opposite.

Here's another case against beer: there is a reason we call big guts 'beer bellies' after all. Beer is loaded with carbs, which, as we've learned, create fat. You don't get off the hook just by switching to low-carb beers; they still have alcohol in them. And alcohol stops your body burning fat. In one study, Swiss researchers gave eight men the equivalent in alcohol of five beers. They found the alcohol slowed the subjects' ability to burn fat by 36 percent.

Here's the chemical process that leads to a beer belly: you take a swig of beer and within seconds, your stomach starts absorbing about 20 percent of the alcohol and sends it directly into your bloodstream. The rest is absorbed in your intestines. The alcohol in your blood is broken down in your liver, where it creates the waste products, acetate and acetaldehyde, which signal your body to stop burning fat. At the same time, your body starts making fat from another waste product of alcohol, acetyl CoA. Double whammy. More fat is made that can't be burned. The same thing happens when you drink wine and spirits such as vodka, gin, and whisky. Spirits contain hardly any carbs, but you'll still get the adverse effects of the alcohol (the cancelling of fat burning, and the storing of waste products as fat). And when you mix spirits with a non-diet fizzy drink or juice, you essentially turn a no-carb

GYM TIP

Burn fat faster by skipping. Ten minutes with the rope will burn the same number of calories as jogging for half an hour. See Chapter Eleven for more rope tricks.

drink into a high-carb drink that'll lead to even more fat storage in your belly. And then, of course, we need to consider our favourite drinking pal: food. (See our Bar Chart, opposite.).

Now, you might be thinking, "What about what I've read on the health benefits of booze?" True, beer and wine contain flavonoids that ward off coronary artery disease, hypertension and even dementia. A substance called resveratrol, found in wine, has been shown to protect the linings of arteries. But doctors say you lose the health benefits of drinking alcohol once you down more than two drinks. You have to ask yourself, how easy is it to limit yourself to just a drink or two at parties or restaurant dinners?

You might, of course, try to be healthier by going for an orange juice down the pub, but that could be even worse. Juice sounds natural and healthy, after all it's rich in vitamin C. But, unless your juice has a lot of pulp, it's like injecting pure sugar directly into your veins. Liquid doesn't have to be broken down as whole fruit does, so the sugar goes directly into the bloodstream. That's why eating fruit is a much smarter option. There's fibre in the skin of an apple and in the white fleshy part of an orange, which slows down the sugar infusion because it takes longer for your intestines to process it. A 2007 study in the *International Journal of Obesity* reported people who substituted a piece of whole fruit for fruit juice with lunch reduced their daily calories by as much as 20 percent. Likewise, when participants ate cheese instead of drinking milk, they saw a similar reduction in calories. Solids take longer to process. What's more, the researchers found the act of chewing stimulates satiety hormones better than swallowing liquid does. If you can't stop drinking juice, buy it with bits in and cut it with water. You'll halve your calories and reduce the blood-sugar rush.

And, of course, we don't need to tell you that drinking a cola or lemonade isn't a recipe for weight-loss success do we? Even diet versions can give you a sweet tooth, making you crave sugar from other sources. So steer clear and go for the best drink of all whenever you can: cool, pure water.

69

The percentage of British men who have at least one drink a day

33

The percentage of British men classed as 'hazardous' drinkers

2.7

The yearly cost, in billions of pounds, of alcohol-related harm

BAR CHART

JUST HOW BAD IS PUB GRUB?

Cutting out alcohol is one of the most effective ways to lose your gut. Why? Because alcohol is high in calories, containing about 7 per gram, which isn't far off the 9 calories you'll find in a gram of fat. But there's another reason to eliminate booze for a month. With beer comes pub grub. It's a fact that when you drink, you want to snack on fatty, salty stuff – from peanuts to pork scratchings. And how many times, after leaving the bar, have you made a pit stop at the kebab shop for a doner with special sauce? Admit it. We've got the videos.

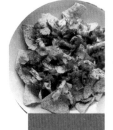

½ bowl nachos with cheese, salsa, sour cream and guacamole

Two pints with . . .

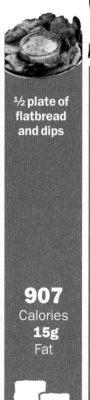

½ plate of flatbread and dips

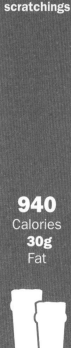

1 bag pork scratchings

1 bowl of chips

1 packet of peanuts

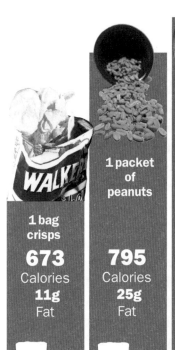

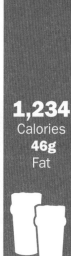

1 bag crisps

673 Calories 11g Fat	**795** Calories 25g Fat	**898** Calories 16g Fat	**907** Calories 15g Fat	**940** Calories 30g Fat	**1,234** Calories 46g Fat

5. Old Father Time Is Against Us

We have much to look forward to as we get older – ear hair, bifocals, a prescription for Viagra. Add a slower metabolism to your list. It's a fact of life – the older you get, the fewer calories you burn. A 12st 12lb (82kg) man in his forties burns on average about 12 fewer calories per hour at rest than a man of the same weight in his twenties. That means he ends the day with 288 more calories than the younger guy – unless he does something about it. Researchers have estimated that the decline continues at the rate of 2-4 percent per decade after age 40. Conspiring to make burning those extra calories even more difficult is the fact that most of us have jobs that don't require physical exertion, especially as we advance in our careers. According to researchers at the University of North Carolina at Wilmington, people who start a typical sedentary office job will gain an average of 1st 2lb (7kg) in the first 8 months.

And while you are burning less energy sitting at that desk, your muscles are shrinking. Between the ages of 30 and 50, the average man loses 6lb (2.7kg) of muscle. No wonder you and your mates at your university reunion looked so different from your graduation pictures. Remember that muscle burns 50 more calories per day than fat does. So when you have less of it, your metabolism slows even more. If you don't scale back your calorie consumption or increase your activity level as you get older, you will gain weight. Guaranteed. And we do. In our 30s and 40s, career and family obligations have a way of making it more difficult for us to find time to take care of our bodies. And often our taste for fine dining and good wine grows over the years, and the opportunities to enjoy both – on the job and socially – increase exponentially.

So now, after reading all this, you may be thinking, "I'm doomed." Human biology and food culture have saddled me with a life-threatening potbelly that's going to be very hard to get rid of.

Don't worry. Understanding how our nation got so fat is a crucial tool to help you sidestep the land mines in your own life. In the next chapter, you'll learn exactly how *The Fat Burner's Bible* works and how you can start to make it part of your healthier lifestyle.

EASY LIFESTYLE TWEAK

If it didn't grow, walk or swim, don't eat it. Processed foods are loaded with unhealthy trans fats and artificial sweeteners.

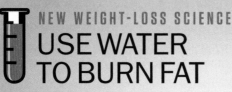

USE WATER TO BURN FAT

Simply holding a bottle of water when you go for a run can help to shift extra pounds. But you need to make sure there's ice in the H_2O; room-temperature won't work. A new study at Stanford University made the surprising discovery by examining overweight women who overheated during exercise. They found holding a bottle of cold water helped them to maintain a low core temperature, increasing endurance. Ultimately, this meant that they ran faster – and burned more fat – than subjects who didn't get cool bottles to hold. As high core temperature is a significant factor for reducing endurance in all athletes, there is no reason why you can't use this trick to counteract it. Its effects will be especially noticeable on hot summer days.

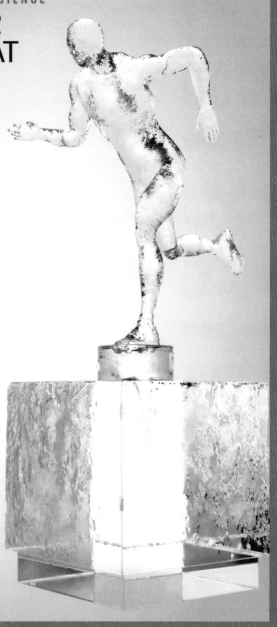

FITNESS

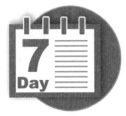

DIARY

7 Day FOOD

A food diary will help you be hyper-aware of what you put in your mouth. It can identify binge triggers and studies show people who write down what they eat lose more weight. Use these pages (or photocopies) and record everything you consume. Try it for at least three days and you'll recognise its power to change habits.

DAY 1

Morning
....
....
....
....
....
....

Lunch
....
....
....
....

Afternoon
....
....
....
....

After 6pm
....
....
....
....
....
....

DAY 2

Morning
....
....
....
....
....
....

Lunch
....
....
....
....

Afternoon
....
....
....
....

After 6pm
....
....
....
....
....
....

DAY 3

Morning
....
....
....
....
....
....

Lunch
....
....
....
....

Afternoon
....
....
....
....

After 6pm
....
....
....
....
....
....

DAY 4

Morning

....
....
....
....
....

Lunch

....
....
....
....

Afternoon

....
....
....
....

After 6pm

....
....
....
....
....

DAY 5

Morning

....
....
....
....
....

Lunch

....
....
....
....

Afternoon

....
....
....
....

After 6pm

....
....
....
....
....

DAY 6

Morning

....
....
....
....
....

Lunch

....
....
....
....

Afternoon

....
....
....
....

After 6pm

....
....
....
....
....

DAY 7

Morning

....
....
....
....
....

Lunch

....
....
....
....

Afternoon

....
....
....
....

After 6pm

....
....
....
....
....

Lewis Ingleby, from Sunderland, filled out on sugary fizzy drinks. Here he reveals how he managed to turn his life around

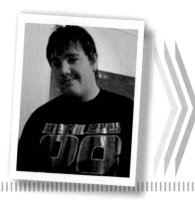

"I HARDLY WALKED, LET ALONE RAN"

Lewis's weight gain began early, although he was active in his youth, nutrition was his Achilles' Heel. "I piled on the weight in my teens, eating sugary cereals and fried food. I wasn't big on booze but I would get through three litres of cola a day." His size made Lewis an imposing presence, but he knew deep down that it didn't count for much. "I was a big bloke, bigger than all of my friends, but none of it was muscle," he says. "Even the thought of entering a gym left me cold, knowing everyone would look at my size and think, 'Why bother, mate?'"

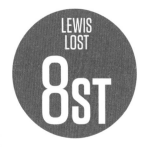

LEWIS LOST

8ST

Ultimately Lewis's weight stopped him from doing the things he loved. "At 21st [133kg] even the sports I enjoyed were out of the question," he says. "I'd never pick myself to play in a team so why would anybody else? I barely walked anywhere, let alone jogged or ran. I even found it difficult to socialise, my confidence was shot to bits and I sought comfort in junk food."

Lewis was given the harshest of wake-up calls when his love life came crashing down around his ears. "My girlfriend dumped me for another bloke, which made me question my appearance, particularly my weight," he says. It was time to do something about it.

SMALL STEPS

"I focused on small goals to give myself a regular sense of achievement," says Lewis. Paul Baard, a sports psychologist at Fordham University, New York, agrees with this methodology: simply relying on the opinions of others (in Lewis's case, his ex girlfriend) isn't usually enough

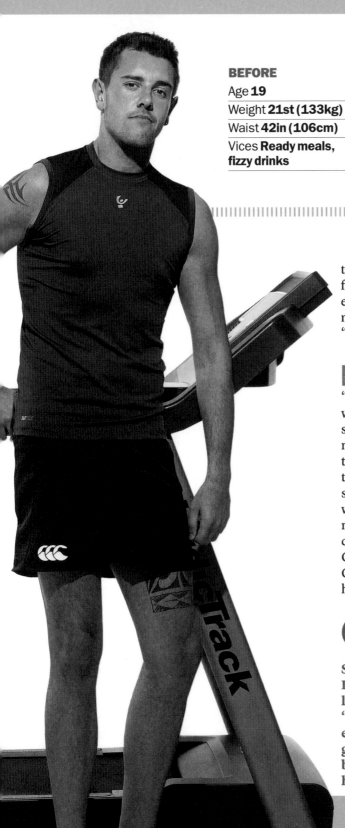

BEFORE	AFTER
Age **19**	Age **21**
Weight **21st (133kg)**	Weight **13st (82kg)**
Waist **42in (106cm)**	Waist **34in (86cm)**
Vices **Ready meals, fizzy drinks**	Victories **Marathon medals, great pics**

to power you though a long-term fitness plan. "Don't make external pressure your sole motivation," says Baard. "Intrinsic motivation is vital."

BIG CHANGES

"I graduated to hill running, which burned extra calories," says Lewis. "And I found that the more I trained, the less I wanted to eat." New research has found that exercise helps to restore the sensitivity of brain neurones which control satiety "Thirty minutes of cardio is enough to control appetite," says Dr José Carvalheira of the University of Campinas, Brazil. For more on his work see Page 36.

 RESULT

Stripping away fat changed Lewis's entire outlook. "My life began again," he says. "I met a new girlfriend who encouraged me to reach my goals, and I'm now toning my body. I'd like to shake my ex's hand for dumping me!"

3

THE
PRINCIPLES
OF THE FAT BURNER'S BIBLE

READING THE PREVIOUS CHAPTER and keeping a food diary should have given you a good idea of the major problems with your diet.

We Brits eat a lot of food. We eat a lot of the wrong kinds of foods – starchy carbs and lots of sugars that go straight to our middles. We eat them at the wrong times of the day – rarely early and mostly late. Sausage and mash with gravy and a bread roll, followed by chocolate cake, for dinner at 8pm. This major infiltration of calories sits there in your belly, while your pancreas works overtime and your thumb works the TV remote. Then you go to sleep, while your digestive system pulls a night shift. Simply put you are taking on more energy than you are expending. What you don't use gets stored as fat.

WHILE IT MAY SEEM THAT THE PRINGLES ARE STACKED AGAINST YOU, there's a way out of this mess. You didn't forget your promise, did you? You've already crossed a huge hurdle even before picking up a fork and lacing-up your running shoes: you've signed the *Fat Burner's Bible* Code of Conduct at the end of Chapter One. It's a commitment to yourself to follow five simple rules. Now we're going to take a look at each one of those in more detail, to explain exactly how they will work, prove how easy they are to follow and explain how you can incorporate them into your life. We'll also take a look at the very latest science, on which they're based. Before we get started, here are those five golden rules of fat-burning again:

 ① Eat a protein-rich breakfast daily

 ② Follow the Bodyweight 100 exercise and intervals programme and start your day with the Two-Minute Drill.

 ③ Eat four to six small meals and snacks a day.

 ④ Eliminate all processed carbs and cut right back on all complex carbs after 6pm. Eat more fruit, veg, protein and a little fat.

 ⑤ Don't drink alcohol for four weeks

There you have it. Eat often throughout the day (and make sure you eat well). Starting with breakfast, cut out empty carbohydrates and get even more strict about this in the evenings. Finally, exercise scientifically. Those are the basic principles of *The Fat Burner's Bible*. Each one of these lifestyle tweaks will ramp up your metabolism, which is your body's fat-burning furnace. Each one has been proven to be successful by the men who've graced the Fat Burner of the Month pages in *Men's Health* magazine over the past 10 years. Each one is easy to stick to for the rest of your life. Follow them religiously for the next four weeks, and you will start to see results – less weight, more energy, fewer cravings – within the first five days of the regime.

Later in this book, you'll learn simple tricks to stick to these rules, plus hundreds of ways to make eating and exercising even more effective at getting rid of belly fat. Here's the science behind the five rules that will help you lose over a stone and half in 30 days.

1. Eat Breakfast

Eating breakfast is like putting kindling on the fire of your metabolism. It's the most important meal of the day. Resolve never to skip the morning meal again. University of Massachusetts Medical School researchers found that men who skip breakfast are 4.5 times more likely to be obese than those who eat it. Try to eat something within 90 minutes of waking up.

"Not eating breakfast may reduce your metabolic rate by up to 10 percent," says Leslie Bonci, a registered dietitian and director of sports nutrition at the University of Pittsburgh Medical Center

Dieters often think they are doing themselves a favour by skipping breakfast. But that strategy can actually sabotage weight-loss efforts. When you don't eat breakfast, you are effectively fasting for 15-20 hours, considering you haven't eaten since dinner and you spent the night sleeping. If you don't break that fast, your body won't produce the enzymes needed to metabolise fat to lose weight. Your body slips into starvation mode, hoarding fat in fear of a famine that never comes. Later in the day when you are ravenous,

EASY LIFESTYLE TWEAK

Don't fool yourself into thinking that 'active' console games like Wii Sports are a subsitute for real exercise. A study published in the *British Medical Journal* found these titles only burn around 2% more calories that traditional computer games. Get out and play real sport instead.

you'll simply open the fridge and stuff your face. Studies show that breakfast skippers tend to replace calories during the day with mindless snacking and they're often so hungry that they'll binge at lunch and dinner.

In a 2008 study, researchers at Virginia Commonwealth University found dieters who ate a protein-rich, 600-calorie breakfast lost significantly more weight in eight months than those who consumed only 300 calories and a quarter of the protein. The big breakfast eaters, who lost nearly 3st (9kg), had an easier time sticking with the diet even though both groups were prescribed about the same number of total daily calories.

Protein at breakfast is clearly important. Another study published in 2008 in the *British Journal of Nutrition* found that eating extra protein for breakfast leads to feelings of fullness that can last throughout the day. The study, conducted by researchers at the University of Kansas Medical Center and Purdue University, scored the feelings of fullness of nine men who were on a regular diet and then while eating a calorie-restricted diet. The results showed that the men on the calorie-restricted diet had their hunger satisfied longest when they ate extra protein at breakfast. "Our findings suggest that people trying to lose weight should eat more protein for breakfast to help them avoid overeating the rest of the day," says study author Dr Heather Leidy, of the University of Kansas Medical Center.

Here's an example of a good high-protein breakfast: have two scrambled eggs, one or two slices of lean bacon, and a 250ml glass of semi-skimmed milk. Top that off with a mid-morning snack of a pot of yoghurt or wholemeal toast with peanut butter.

Don't be afraid of a little saturated fat, either. If you're healthy, there's no scientific reason that natural foods containing saturated fat can't be part of your diet. However, the kind of breakfast outlined above does take time to prepare – time you may not have in the morning. So when you're rushed, slather some peanut butter on a banana, eat a protein bar or roll a slice of turkey in a slice of Swiss cheese. Leave a bowl of fruit or bags of trail mix near your front

Get outside for your workout. The University of Barcelona found exercising in direct sunlight increased fat-burning by as much as 20 percent. This was linked with a boost in the production of appetite-killing hormone leptin.

door so you can grab them as you leave for work in the morning. Even cold pizza can be breakfast in a real emergency, just, whatever you do, don't skip this meal.

2. Work Out

Study after study has shown that dieting alone rarely works, and weight loss is impossible to sustain without some exercise. That's why we're making it part of your daily morning routine, like shaving and letting the dog out. *The Fat Burner's Bible* Two-Minute Drill, a circuit detailed in Chapter Four, is designed to start your day off on the right foot. It sparks your fat-burners after a night of sleep and serves as an alarm bell to remind you that the key to weight loss is keeping your metabolism high all day long. Plus, studies have shown that athletes who work out first thing in the morning stoke their metabolisms higher and longer and burn more calories throughout the day than those who did their workouts at the end of the day.

Ideally, use The Two-Minute Drill as a warm-up to a full morning workout – and then you'll be done for the day. But if you can't find time for a full workout in the morning, that's okay. Just do the drill when you wake up, and do your longer workout in the afternoon or evening. What's critical is that you fit in three or four bodyweight routines per week and two or three workouts of high-intensity interval training. As mentioned earlier, the combination of muscle-building moves and cardio-enhancing intervals has a powerful effect on belly fat. Skeletal muscle burns more calories than fat does, so it serves you to add muscle mass.

When it comes to cardio, new research shows that intervals – short bursts of intense exertion interspersed with periods of slower activity – burn fat and improve fitness more quickly than long, moderate bouts of exercise. And intervals trigger an afterburn effect similar to weight lifting, keeping your body churning through calories long after you've finished in the shower. In a study by a researcher in the Department of Human Health and

EASY LIFESTYLE TWEAK

Use a pedometer. Studies have shown that men who wore pedometers to log their daily step boosted their activity levels by 16 percent.

Nutritional Sciences at the University of Guelph in Canada, exercisers were asked to ride an exercise bike every other day for two weeks. They alternated between 10 sets of four-minute bursts of riding at 90 percent effort with two-minute slow-pedalling rest intervals. Researcher Jason Talanian found that the subjects experienced an increase in fat used during the intervals as well as an increase in a muscle enzyme that burns fat. What's more, after interval training, the amount of fat the subjects burned in an hour of even moderate pedaling also increased by 36 percent. So intense intervals had the effect of turbocharging even easy-level exercise. Make sure you build some into your regime.

3. Eat Regularly

Eat three meals and one or two snacks every day to keep your metabolism well stoked and therefore working at optimum speed, a typical eating timetable might look something like the chart below. A study in the *American Journal of Epidemiology* found men who ate this frequently were half as likely to become overweight compared with men who ate just three or fewer times daily. Spacing your calories throughout the day by eating something every three hours or so keeps blood sugar levels even and controls the release of insulin that can cause your body to store more calories as fat. When you eat less frequently or skip meals, your metabolic furnace goes cold, triggering your body's primal instinct to slow down, conserve energy and store fat. By contrast, every time you eat, your metabolism speeds up as it swings into action to digest the food.

Whenever possible, prepare your own meals from raw ingredients. This way you will reduce your need to visit fast-food shops or resort to readymeals, which are often high in calories, carbs, salt and fat. Cooking your own food gives you a proper understanding of exactly what it is you are eating at each and every meal.

6:30 A.M.	› BREAKFAST
10:00 A.M.	› SNACK
1:00 P.M.	› LUNCH
4:00 P.M.	› SNACK
6:30 P.M.	› DINNER
8:30 P.M.	› SNACK (OPTIONAL)

4. Cut Refined Carbs

 To follow *The Fat Burner's Bible* meal plan it is crucial to eliminate or cut back drastically on cakes, biscuits, chocolate, fizzy drinks, fruit juice, white bread, pasta, potatoes and sugary breakfast cereals. All of these are fast-absorbing, refined carbohydrates, the foods that spike blood sugar, instigate cravings and help fat set up residence round your middle. Remember, nearly all *Men's Health* Fat Burners used this strategy to lose their guts. Dozens of studies support restricting carbs to force your body to burn fat. If you're not sure about a product, simply check the ingredients: skip those that contain sugar – often listed as sucrose, glucose-fructose, or cane syrup – and refined flour, which is any flour that doesn't start with the word 'whole' (as in wholemeal).

Refined carbs are easily digested so, if you don't use the energy they contain immediately, your body will store it as fat. This is why it's particularly bad to eat large amounts of carbohydrate in the evening: you simply don't have time to burn it off before bed. What's more a recent study at the University of California at Davis found keeping carbs to less than 40 percent of your total daily calories actually deactivates a gene that produces triglycerides – the blood fats that collect as body fat. You should automatically achieve it just by following the basic guidelines and recipes in this book.

However, it's also important to remember that slow-burning complex carbohydrates are essential to good health. So replace highly processed foods in your diet with vegetables and whole fruits, wholemeal bread, brown rice and pasta. These foods are also rich in fibre, "the best thing you can eat when you are trying to lose weight," says Gay Riley, a registered dietitian. Fibre binds with other foods to help hustle calories out of the body and because they slow your rate of digestion, they keep you feeling full longer and reduce cravings for more food.

Check out the tips on page 176 for some easy ways of getting more fibre in your diet. If you still need a little extra help getting enough you can actually buy it in supplement form. Metamucil is

EASY LIFESTYLE TWEAK

Don't go shopping hungry. Instead of getting a few essentials, you'll end up buying the whole aisle. Stick to a list and shop when you're full – you'll think more about what you're buying than what would be most tasty.

HIT OR MYTH?

BURN MORE FAT BY MAXIMISING ENERGY LEVELS (OR NOT)

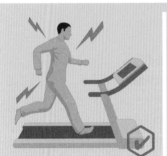

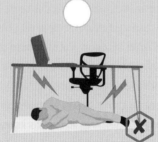

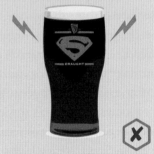

You start slowly in the mornings

The early bird might catch the worm, but you have more chance of burning more fat at night than in the morning. Your peak performance will normally be around 11pm, says University of South Carolina research. Our circadian rhythms impact athletic performance. Ideal if you need to run for the last bus.

The afternoon slump is all about blood-sugar

Blood sugar is behind other power cuts but there's something deeper at work here. "It's likely you're low on serotonin, which makes you feel alert," says Judith Wurtman, a researcher at Massachusetts Institute of Technology. Snack on cheese or turkey, both are rich in tryptophan, which your body needs to produce serotonin.

Always tired? You need more vitamins

Supplements that say they'll increase energy are usually B vitamins or iron. Both found in Guinness, incidentally. B vitamins help release energy from food, so deficiency causes tiredness. "Most of us get enough," says Dr Connie Diekman, director of nutrition at Washington University. "So taking more won't do anything."

available at astronutrition.com for £27.99 for 30 capsules. You dissolve it in a glass of water and drink it about 5 minutes before you eat a meal. The psyllium fibre binds to the food you eat, making it slower to digest. In essence, it lowers the Glycaemic Load of your meal.

In addition to cutting carbs and increasing fibre, the *Fat Burner's Bible* eating plan also encourages you to consume protein and fat with every meal. Fat because it is satiating. It adds satisfying flavour to foods and it makes you feel as if you have eaten something substantial. Protein because it is your strongest ally in the war against a big belly. Here's why...

Protein makes you feel full quicker and it takes about two hours longer than carbs to digest, so you won't get hungry as soon. It takes more energy for your body to digest protein than it does for it to digest carbohydrates or fat. "Protein burns hotter than other food sources," says Dr Mark Hyman, author of *Ultrametabolism.* So the more protein you eat, the more calories you'll burn in the process of digestion. A British study found that people who increased the percentage of calories from protein in their meals burned 71 more calories per day than people on low-protein diets. (That amounts to 7.4 pounds of fat lost per year.)

Protein also accelerates muscle growth and speeds your recovery after vigorous exercise by helping to rebuild stressed muscle fibres. How much protein you should get depends upon your level of activity. If you're working out regularly you need to aim for roughly 1g of protein for every two pounds of body weight (or roughly 1g for every kg). Terrific sources of protein are lean meats and fish and other animal products, such as eggs, milk, and cheese. One hundred grams of chicken breast, for example, contains about 30 grams of protein. You can also get your protein from beans, lentils, nuts, and seeds. One hundred grams of kidney beans or chickpeas contains about 7g of protein, while the same amount of tofu has over 10g.

5. Avoid Alcohol

If you are a guy who enjoys a couple of beers every night, some wine with dinner, and maybe margaritas on the weekends, cutting out alcohol will give you an enormous head start on shedding pounds and belly fat. Abstain for a month and you'll be convinced. Alcohol stops your body from burning fat and depending upon what you drink (beer or cocktails made with sugary mixers) it can be loaded with a lot of 'empty' carbs which will fill you out without filling you up. Cutting booze of all types for just four weeks is the best way to start controlling your sugar intake. It won't be forever. Just four weeks. You can do it.

EASY LIFESTYLE TWEAK

When you do start drinking again, switch to spirits. A single gin and slimline tonic has just 56 calories but a pint of Stella contains 250.

THE FAT BURNER'S
LABEL DECODER
HOW TO USE FOOD PACKAGING TO FAST-TRACK WEIGHT LOSS

IT HAS BEEN LAW for many years in the UK that all packaged food must carry nutritional information. However, in order to combat the growing problem of obesity, the government took action in 1998 and collaborated with the food industry to develop a system of Guideline Daily Amounts (GDAs), which typically appear on the front of packaging. While it is not law for all foods to use this system, many manufacturers now adopt it. A third system is Recommended Daily Amounts (RDA), which are set by the European Union to give guidelines for vitamin and mineral intake.

   Over the next three pages we look at all three types of label. Understanding food packaging will help you eat the right foods to fast-track your fat burning.

RECOMMENDED DAILY ALLOWANCE
OUTLINING YOUR SUGGESTED MICRONUTRIENT INTAKE

Let's start small. Recommended Daily Allowances (RDAs) are set by the European Food Information Council and focus on vitamins and minerals that, although tiny in their volume, are essential to the proper functioning of our bodies. We must get them in our diet as our bodies cannot synthesise these themselves. The exact amounts required have been developed by compiling scientific studies on the levels needed to maintain a healthy body, but some people may require more, particularly if they are very active.

   It's important to note that whereas GDA (overleaf) is all about maximum levels, RDA is based on minimum requirements. Getting even as much as five times your RDA of vitamin C, for example, won't cause you harm, whereas five times your GDA for salt or saturated fat is an entirely different matter.

   One-a-day multivitamin tablets usually contain 100% of the RDA of the most important nutrients, but it's easy to get 100% of your RDA if you eat a balanced diet. Check out the chart on the next page to ensure you're eating right.

YOUR BEST VITAMIN AND MINERAL SOURCES

ZINC
Sources Meat, dairy products
Uses Making new cells, healing wounds and injuries
100% = 100g dark chocolate

VITAMIN A
Sources Oily fish, eggs, yoghurt
Uses Helps strengthen immune system, vision and skin
100% = 150g sweet potato or carrots

B1 THIAMIN
Sources Oats, rice, cauliflower
Uses Helps release energy from foods – essential for nervous system.
100% = 150g grilled lean pork chop

POTASSIUM
Sources Potatoes, bananas
Uses Brain function, restful sleep,
100% = 2 large melons

B2 RIBOFLAVIN
Sources Asparagus, popcorn
Uses Helps with growth of skin and with energy release from protein and carbs.
100% = 1½ pints milk

CALCIUM
Sources Milk, leafy green veg, nuts, soya
Uses Strong teeth and bones, muscle regulation
100% = ¾ pot natural yoghurt

B3 NIACIN
Sources Dates, broccoli, tuna
Uses Helps control blood sugar levels and energy release.
100% = one chicken breast

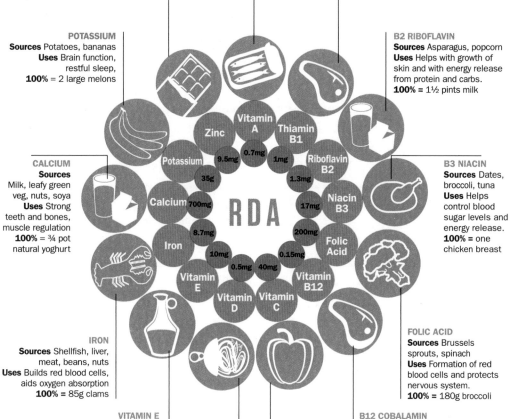

Zinc
Vitamin A
Thiamin B1
Riboflavin B2
Niacin B3
Folic Acid
Vitamin B12
Vitamin C
Vitamin D
Vitamin E
Iron
Calcium
Potassium

RDA

9.5mg
0.7mg
1mg
1.3mg
35g
700mg
17mg
8.7mg
200mg
10mg
0.15mg
0.5mg
40mg

IRON
Sources Shellfish, liver, meat, beans, nuts
Uses Builds red blood cells, aids oxygen absorption
100% = 85g clams

FOLIC ACID
Sources Brussels sprouts, spinach
Uses Formation of red blood cells and protects nervous system.
100% = 180g broccoli

VITAMIN E
Sources Olive oil, nuts and seeds
Uses Protects cell membranes
100% = 50g hazelnuts

B12 COBALAMIN
Sources Liver, milk, eggs
Uses Blood cell and nerve function
100% = 100g sirloin steak

VITAMIN D
Sources Oily fish, eggs, tuna
Uses Regulates calcium, helps to build strong bones
100% = 15 minutes direct sunlight

VITAMIN C
Sources Peppers, broccoli, oranges
Uses Helps formation of cells, connective tissue and boosts immunity
100% = 1 kiwi fruit

GUIDELINE DAILY AMOUNTS

HELPS YOU AVOID EXCESS NUTRIENTS THAT COULD BE HARMFUL

Each pack contains:

Calories	Sugars	Fat	Saturates	Salt
183	0.2g	11.7g	0.9g	0.5g
9%	<1%	17%	5%	8%

of an adult's guideline daily amount

CALORIES

This shows the number of calories in a serving along with the percentage that this is of your GDA. It's worth noting that this is based on a woman's recommended 2,000kcal a day. Men can consumer more like 2,500kcal. Nevertheless this provides useful at-a-glance information for all.

Each pack contains:

Calories	Sugars	Fat	Saturates	Salt
183	**0.2g**	11.7g	0.9g	0.5g
9%	**<1%**	17%	5%	8%

of an adult's guideline daily amount

SUGARS

Sugar is a useful instant fuel for the body, but if it's not used quickly it gets turned to fat, so it is important to keep an eye on your intake. Again, labels like this express this value as a percentage of a woman's GDA. Women should have no more than 90g, for a man it's 120g.

Each pack contains:

Calories	Sugars	Fat	Saturates	Salt
183	0.2g	**11.7g**	0.9g	0.5g
9%	<1%	**17%**	5%	8%

of an adult's guideline daily amount

FAT

Fats get a bad rap, but are critical for a whole host of bodily functions, particularly the unsaturated type and essential omega-3s. Nevertheless, too much can be harmful. A man can have up to 95g a day, whereas a woman can only have 70g (the percentage of which is expressed here).

Each pack contains:

Calories	Sugars	Fat	Saturates	Salt
183	0.2g	11.7g	**0.9g**	0.5g
9%	<1%	17%	**5%**	8%

of an adult's guideline daily amount

SATURATES

These fats are linked with heart disease and should be avoided whenever possible. However, it's not that easy as they're in everything from meat to cakes. As men we can get away with 30g, 50% higher than the woman's GDA of 20g, which is the one you'll find on this label.

Each pack contains:

Calories	Sugars	Fat	Saturates	Salt
183	0.2g	11.7g	0.9g	**0.5g**
9%	<1%	17%	5%	**8%**

of an adult's guideline daily amount

SALT

The GDA of salt for a man is the same as it is for a woman, so the percentages shown on food packets are always spot on. A large amount of salt can lead to high blood pressure, but in small amounts are important for muscle function. You should never have more than 6g a day.

NUTRITIONAL INFORMATION

GIVES YOU THE FULL BREAKDOWN OF EVERYTHING IN A PRODUCT

Nutritional Information		
Typical Values	30g	100g
1 Energy	370kJ	1230kJ
	90kcal	290kcal
2 Protein	0.9g	3.0g
3 Carbohydrate	20.2g	67.3g
4 of which sugars	17.4g	58.1g
5 Fat	0.2g	0.7g
of which saturates	0.1g	0.3g
6 Fibre	0.2g	0.7g
7 Sodium	Trace	Trace
Salt Equivalent	Trace	Trace

SUGAR

4 The most refined type of carb, so it's easily digested and converted to energy (or fat). As such it is easy to have too much of it. See GDA for recommended limits.

FAT

5 Some fat is essential, but saturated fat is linked with health problems such as high blood pressure and heart disease. Again, keep within your GDA.

FIBRE

6 Useful for a healthy gut and for aiding digestion. Fibre helps with weight loss by increasing feelings of fullness. You should aim to get around 5g in every meal or snack.

ENERGY

1 Energy is shown in calories (kcal) and kilojoules (kJ). Be careful not to muddle them up. These figures show how much energy is in a food, but not how easy it is for your body to digest, so they can be misleading; particulary if you are comparing carbs with fat.

PROTEIN

2 Protein is important for repairing damaged cells and building muscle. If you are following the workouts in this book you need to make sure you are getting some at every meal, and also directly after a workout. Around 20g is a decent serving.

CARBOHYDRATE

3 Carbohydrates are your body's preferred source of energy as they are easy to break down. Even a small amount of calories in carb form can be quickly turned into energy. Try to limit yourself to no more than 20g after 6pm in the evening.

SALT

7 High levels of salt can contribute to high blood pressure and too much can ultimately lead to heart attacks, so never have more than 6g a day. However, a little salt is useful for aiding nerve action, regulating body fluid levels and preventing muscle cramp.

HOW TO TELL GOOD FATS FROM BAD

DOCTORS AND NUTRITIONISTS have been warning us about the dangers of fat for years. An entire health industry has sprouted from the idea that fat is bad. Yet, while statistics show our fat intake has been dropping, the number of fat Britons has been rising.

One reason, many experts agree, is that we are eating more calories than ever before, thanks to fat-free foods. Less fat equals less guilt equals more eating. Some doctors have even suggest that if we weren't so anal about eating fat, we'd all be a lot thinner.

While being less vigilant about dietary fat is an appealing notion it is still important to be clear about the total amount of fat that you eat and remember that it's high in calories and those calories still matter. Even more important is understanding the type of fat that you eat. Here's how to tell your saturates from your omega-3s

Saturated Fats

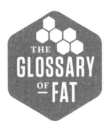

You find them mainly in meats, butter, cheese and eggs. Some raise your low-density lipoprotein (LDL) or "bad" cholesterol, and increase your risk of heart disease and stroke. But a growing number of researchers believe the real culprit is consuming too many calories and carbs. The message is not to gorge on butter and bacon, but that there's no scientific evidence to suggest that natural foods containing saturated fat shouldn't be a part of a healthy diet. The Food and Drink Federation, who developed the UK's Guideline Daily Amounts (GDA), recommends a man of average weight eats no more than 30g of saturated fat a day.

Trans Fats

They're in biscuits, cakes, hot dogs and pretty much anything deep fried. A trans fat is created when hydrogen is added to vegetable oil to keep it "stable" for frying (unstable oil makes food taste bad) and to stop it from going rancid. They're what makes a half-eaten mini roll you found under your sofa look as new as it did when your nephew hid it there a year ago.

THE GLOSSARY OF FAT

Avoid at all costs

Limit your intake

Seek these out

Trans fats are, for the most part, manufactured fats. In order to remove cholesterol from their products, makers of processed foods have been replacing saturated fats (such as lard and beef tallow) with hydrogenated vegetable oils. They take vegetable oil, heat it to high temperatures, and pump in hydrogen, which bonds with the oil molecules to create a new form of fat that stays solid at room temperature. This is ideal for makers of biscuits, cakes, muffins, waffles, chocolate bars and fish sticks, who need oil in a solid form to make their products taste good and look appealing. The words "hydrogenated" or "partially hydrogenated" on the ingredients list will tip you off to the trans fats.

Trans fat should be aggressively avoided because of its unhealthy effect on your cholesterol levels – increasing LDL cholesterol and lowering the "good" high-density lipoprotein (HDL) cholesterol. Trans fat has also appears to damage cells lining blood vessels, leading to inflammation.

Though the dangers of trans fat have been highly publicised, it's easy to forget about them when you've had several pints and the takeaway with its deep-fried delights is calling. Even if you do remember the warnings there's never an ingredients list to check. Instead stick to this rule: if it doesn't look natural, it probably isn't

Monounsaturated Fats

You'll find these in olive, canola, and peanut oils. Studies show that these fats can also help you burn fat. And because they're digested slowly, they make you feel fuller longer. These fats are also considered "heart healthy," because they either have no effect on cholesterol levels or, in the form of oleic acid, lower LDL cholesterol without affecting HDL cholesterol.

Polyunsaturated Fats

These are found in corn, safflower, soybean, and sunflower oils. Unlike monos, polys lower both good and bad cholesterol (LDL and HDL). But animal research has shown that a type of polyunsaturated fat called conjugated linoleic

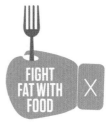

FIGHT FAT WITH FOOD

Cook with fresh onions. "They contain oils and minerals that help break down fat deposits and speed up your metabolism," says nutritionist Sarah Reilly. "They also have thermogenic activity, which helps create heat in your body, which in turns helps burn calories"

acid, CLA for short, found in certain meats and dairy products, may have strong health benefits – including reducing abdominal fat, protecting against heart disease and diabetes, and inhibiting the growth of prostate cancer cells.

Essential Fatty Acids

Omega-6 and omega-3 fatty acids are the two basic ones; they fall under the polyunsaturated fats umbrella. We get more omega-6s than we need from cooking oils, meat, eggs and dairy products, but not nearly enough omega-3s, which are found in certain types of fish and in walnuts, flaxseed and green leafy vegetables. Focus on getting more omega-3s. The richest sources are oily fish like sardines, mackerel, tuna and salmon. If you don't like fish take a fish-oil supplement instead.

Omega-3s are important because they slow the body's production of prostaglandins – chemicals that can cause excessive blood clotting, which can lead to heart attacks. In addition, omega-3s are thought to influence your metabolism, determining whether you burn calories or store them as fat, by altering levels of a hormone called leptin in your body. Studies have found a correlation between low levels of leptin and a faster metabolism. In research at the University of South Australia's Nutritional Physiology Research Centre, overweight men were assigned to one of two groups. One group ate tuna or took fish oil and did aerobic exercise, the other group took sunflower oil and also exercised. At the end of 12 weeks, the exercisers who consumed omega-3s reduced their body fat and improved their metabolic and cardiovascular health. The sunflower oil sippers experienced no such benefit, but their breath smelled a whole lot better.

Now on to seeds and nuts. You know what a walnut is, so let's give a quick shout out to flaxseed, a powerful, but often overlooked superfood. This stuff, which looks like shiny brown sesame seeds, is packed with omega-3s plus cholesterol-fighting fibre. They're also pretty versatile. You can sprinkle them on breakfast cereal, toss them into soups and stew, even use them in spaghetti with

GYM TIP

A study at Temple University found taking a creatine supplement after resistance training will increase your body's metabolic rate by 6% – so you'll burn more fat.

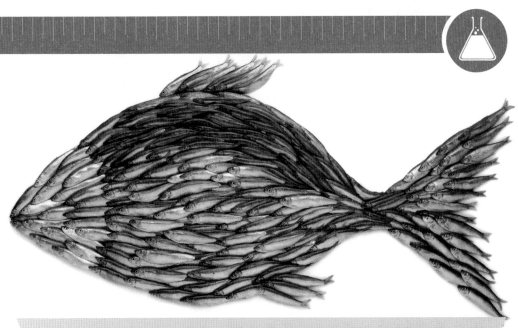

HERE'S THE CATCH

THE TOP 10 BEST SEAFOODS FOR OMEGA-3S

The average Brit eats about 15lb (7kg) of fish a year. But most of that comes battered and deep fried with chips, mushy peas and tartar sauce – all loaded with fat, salt, and calories. You can do much better by choosing fish that's high in omega-3 fats and having it steamed, grilled or baked. Here are the specifications on the best of the best, according to the Cleveland Clinic in the US. All are based on a small 85g serving.

FISH*	OMEGA-3 CONTENT
Herring	1.9g
Sardines	1.5g
Tuna	1.5g
Mackerel	1.5g
Salmon	1.0g
Swordfish	0.9g
Sea bass	0.65g
Tuna (white meat), canned	0.5g
Jumbo shrimp (6 pieces)	0.15g
Lobster	0.15g

tomato sauce. They've got a pleasant, nutty flavour, so they're also excellent mixed into yogurt or sprinkled on top of ice cream. Buy a bag online and have it deli; they're available whole or ground. You might also find flaxseed at your supermarket as grocers become hip to this trendy seed.

Mike Hare from Cambridgeshire survived a car crash that made him reassess his life and inspired him to lose weight, big time...

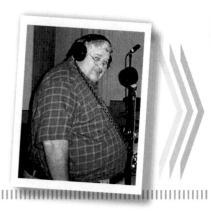

"I THOUGHT I WAS GOING TO DIE"

Mike's life was in a rut. He had been steadily gaining weight over his entire life until, by the age of 50, he was so big he struggled to walk to the local shop – he'd get in his car and drive instead. Then he got the wake-up call he needed to turn his life around – a serious road traffic accident. "I was lucky to survive," says Mike. "I had a second chance at life and asked my GP to help me lose weight. He gave me pills, but the side-effects made me seek out natural alternatives."

Mike started a blog about his weight-loss progress, called 'The Incredible Shrinking Man.' He quickly built up a following, and found that the encouraging words of others helped to keep him motivated.

EAT THIS, NOT THAT

Mike's first step was to overhaul his nutrition. "I swapped my favourite dinner – the McDonald's Big Tasty – for chicken stir-fries with veg and brown rice." Using brown rice instead of white will give you 10 times the fibre, leaving you fuller for longer. "And I only snacked on fruit," says Mike. Natural sugars in fruit help to satisfy cravings without filling you out. And when Mike needed energy for running, he cooked his pasta *al dente* (so it was still slightly hard). Cooking pasta for longer breaks down its sugars, causing an insulin spike that makes you feel hungrier, sooner.

EVERYDAY EXERCISE

"I started jogging to the shops, not driving," says Mike. "Soon I was running." Before buying running shoes, see a specialist.

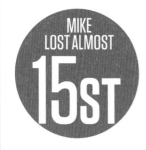

MIKE LOST ALMOST **15ST**

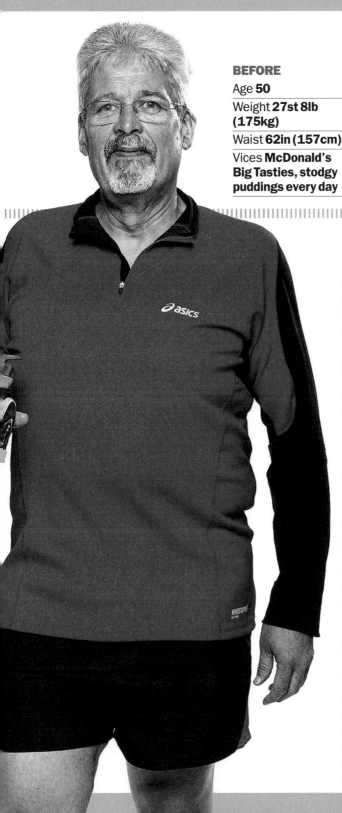

BEFORE		AFTER
Age **50**		Age **54**
Weight **27st 8lb (175kg)**		Weight **12.7st (79.4kg)**
Waist **62in (157cm)**		Waist **37in (93cm)**
Vices **McDonald's Big Tasties, stodgy puddings every day**		Victories **Marathon medals, boosted confidence**

If you're overweight you're 30% more likely to over-pronate, and risk injury. "I mixed up running to include hill work, distance and recovery runs," says Mike. "At the gym I did reclining bike and rower on resistance level five." Do a morning run, too. You're in a 'fasting' state, as you haven't replaced carbs burned overnight – so you'll burn more fat.

A NEW LIFE

Mike's transformation from a 27st fast-food lover to a 12st athlete is an inspiration to anyone who thinks getting fit is beyond them. Mike more than halved his bodyweight and now competes in marathons. If he can do it, you can, too.

 RESULT

"After hundreds of miles running competitive races and shedding 15st, I've written a book about my experience," says Mike, who still runs every day, and gets to the shops quicker, too.

(4)

HOW TO
LOSE WEIGHT
IN ONE WEEK

> **YOUR SEVEN-DAY QUICK-START
> GUIDE TO FIGHTING FLAB**

THINK BACK TO WHEN YOU WERE A TEENAGER sleeping until noon on a Saturday after a late night. Did your parents ever shout at you to get out of bed? Maybe then they set you to work on a few chores?

If they did then, believe it or not, they were actually teaching you important life lessons. Ones that will be useful as you embark on this weight-loss regime. The truth is that a kick up the backside is a good thing now and then, even if you're not a teenager anymore. Having a plan of action is even better. The next seven days are designed to give you both of those things. Follow it to the letter and you'll be starting next week that bit thinner than you are now.

quick start

TO MAKE *THE FAT BURNER'S BIBLE* easy to incorporate into your life, we've listed the steps you'll need to take during this first week. There's only three of them, so there's no excuse for missing any out. You don't have to think. Just follow them and you'll get the picture by Friday. Before you start, though, you need to have read the chapters that come before this one. You also need to have filled out the food diary at the end of Chapter Two for at least a few days. Done that? Good. Let's get started...

STEP 1 With your food diary in hand, clean out your fridge and cupboards, paying particular attention to the bad stuff your diary identified. Dump any pastas, cereals or breads that aren't 100 percent wholemeal and any non-diet fizzy drinks.

STEP 2 Copy the Week One Shopping List opposite, take it to the supermarket and stock up. Everything you need to eat for the first week is on the list. Follow the week's meal plan to the letter. (Use the recipes and cooking instructions where needed.) Don't worry. You're going to love this food. It's man food. It tastes great. It's designed to control calories, saturated fat and carbs, while energizing your body with metabolism-revving fuel. Eating this way for just one week will eliminate guesswork. You can tailor your weekly meal plans to your specific tastes later on.

STEP 3 Follow the exercise schedule outlined on page 79. The descriptions of the workouts and exercises not in this chapter can be found in Chapter Five. By knowing how you are going to exercise every day and what you're going to eat, you'll be more likely to make this quick-start a ritual.

A New Way Of Eating

Using the shopping list opposite it should be easy to fill your fridge with fat-busting foods. If the list looks at bit long, and the cost of your shop goes up, there's a reason. Better, fresher foods generally cost more than processed, packaged foods. But using this guide you can rest assured that nothing will go to waste as you'll also be using leftovers cleverly at every opportunity.

WEEK ONE SHOPPING LIST

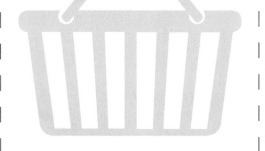

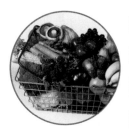

FRUIT, VEGETABLES AND FRESH HERBS

- 1 tin chopped tomatoes
- 1 jar roasted red peppers
- 1 small fresh pepper
- 2 onions
- 1 iceberg lettuce
- 1 bag baby spinach
- 1 bunch celery
- 1 punnet cherry tomatoes
- 2 tomatoes
- 1 tub sundried tomatoes
- A few fresh black olives
- 2 avocados
- 1 bunch asparagus
- 1 packet green beans
- 1 bag carrots
- 2 heads of broccoli
- 2 bunches red grapes
- 1 large punnet blueberries
- 5 apples
- 4 bananas
- 2 fresh chillies
- 1 bulb garlic

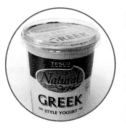

DAIRY AISLE

- Large pot low-fat natural yoghurt
- 4 pints skimmed milk
- 150ml low-fat sour cream
- 250g low-fat cheddar cheese
- 1 tub light cream cheese
- 1 box Dairylea Triangles
- 1 block low-fat feta
- 1 box eggs

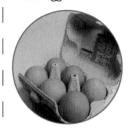

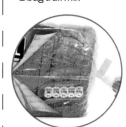

BEANS, NUTS, RICE

- 1 tin kidney beans
- 1 bag raw almonds
- 1 bag trail mix

BREAD, CEREAL, PASTA

- 1 loaf wholemeal bread
- 1 box Kellogg's All-Bran
- 1 box oat cakes
- 500g wholemeal pasta
- 1 pack wholemeal tortillas

MEATS AND FISH

- 10 rashers lean bacon
- 2 salmon fillets
- 200g turkey mince (or extra-lean beef mince)
- 400g cooked turkey breast
- 2 chicken breasts
- 100g cooked prawns
- 2 sea bass fillets

DIPS, CONDIMENTS & DESSERTS

- Hot salsa
- Natural peanut butter
- Light mayonnaise
- 1 tub light coleslaw
- 300g tub of hummus
- 1 tub lemon sorbet

SPICES AND STORE CUPBOARD ITEMS

- Hot chilli powder
- Black pepper
- Sea salt
- Olive oil
- Balsamic vinegar
- Green tea bags
- Regular tea bags
- Coffee

YOUR REAL-MEAL MENU FOR WEEK ONE

	Monday	Tuesday	Wednesday
7 am **Breakfast**	• 2 eggs, scrambled • 2 slices lean bacon • 1 slice wholemeal toast, peanut butter • 1 apple • Tea or coffee • Water	• 1 bowl of All Bran with skimmed milk • 1 banana • Tea or coffee • Water	• Hot Breakfast Burrito (recipe page 143) • 2 slices lean bacon • Tea or coffee • Water
10 am **Morning Snack**	• 1 banana • 2 Dairylea Triangles • Water	• Celery sticks with low-fat cream cheese • Water	• Handful blueberries • 250g low-fat yogurt • Water
1:30 pm **Lunch**	• Turkey, roasted red pepper and salad sandwich • Tea or water	• Mediterranean Wrap (recipe page 144) • 1 apple • Green tea	• Leftover chilli • ½ pot low-fat coleslaw • Green tea
4 pm **Afternoon Snack**	• A few red grapes • 30g almonds • Water	• Handful blueberries • 30g cheddar • Water	• 30g almonds • 2 Dairylea triangles • Green tea
7 pm **Dinner**	• Spicy Sea Bass (recipe page 154) • Grilled Asparagus • Red grapes • Green tea	• Easy Chilli (recipe page 157) • ½ pot low-fat coleslaw • Tea or water	• Spicy Sea Bass (repeat recipe from Monday) • Carrots and broccoli (steamed) • Water
9 pm **Evening Snack** **(optional)**	• Handful trail mix	• Sorbet	• Handful red grapes

Thursday	Friday	Saturday	Sunday
• Lean bacon sandwich • 1 apple • Tea or coffee • Water	• 1 bowl of All Bran with skimmed milk • 1 banana • 2 oat cakes with peanut butter • Tea or Coffee	• Hot Breakfast Burrito (recipe page 143) • 1 apple • Tea or coffee • Water	• 1 bowl of All Bran with skimmed milk • 1 banana • 2 oat cakes with peanut butter • Tea or coffee • Water
• 2 Dairylea Triangles • Handful blueberries • Water	• 30g almonds • 1 apple • Water	• Handful blueberries • 250g low-fat yogurt • Water	• 1 apple with peanut butter
• Peanut butter sandwich on wholemeal • Tea or water	• Prawn and Pasta Salad (recipe page 145) • Green tea	• Bacon, lettuce, and tomato sandwich on wholemeal toast with low-fat mayonnaise • Tea or water	• Leftover Prawn and Pasta Salad (from Friday) • Green tea
• Raw carrot slices • Hummus dip • Water	• Two Dairylea Triangles • Handful trail mix • Water	• Raw baby carrots • Hummus dip • Water	• Celery sticks • Low-fat cream cheese • Water
• Grilled salmon • Broccoli and green beans (steamed) • Red grapes • Green tea	• Greek Style Stuffed Chicken (recipe page 156) • Garden salad • Red grapes	• Grilled salmon • Garden salad • Red grapes • Green tea	• Greek Style Stuffed Chicken (use leftovers from Friday) • Broccoli and carrots (steamed) • Water
• Handful trail mix	• Green tea • Sorbet	• Handful grapes	• Handful trail mix

THE FAT BURNER'S TWO-MINUTE DRILL

Now you've got your eating plan in place, you need to think about your exercise regime. One of the secrets of burning fat in just one week is the Two-Minute Drill.

Why do you usually try to schedule your doctor's visit for the first appointment of the day? To get in and out fast and avoid the waiting-room time suck (and those blue-haired ladies). Why is it best to take the first flight out in the morning? Because airport delays are more likely as the day progresses. For the same reason, you want to get some exercise at the start of the day, because the day's events can conspire to destroy your best-laid plans.

The Two-Minute Drill jump-starts your metabolism, revving it up as soon as you wake up so you'll burn fat more efficiently all day. Exercise in the morning also helps to wake you up, bringing oxygen to your brain and triggering your body to release feel-good hormones. Plus, it starts your day on a positive note. Even if the rest of your day is a complete disaster, you will have still broken a sweat.

So make the Two-Minute Drill part of your morning routine. In a matter of weeks, it'll become so natural it'll seem awkward to skip, like walking out the door without brushing your teeth. Perform the circuit over the page every morning. Do each exercise for 15 seconds, then move immediately to the next until you have done all eight in just two minutes.

What If You Find The Drill Too Difficult?

The Drill will get anyone huffing and puffing. It's a morning jump start. But it may not be for everyone. If you are heavy or have been sedentary for a long time or if you find one of the eight exercises painful or too difficult, change the drill to suit your situation. Remember: the purpose is to get your body moving and kick-start your metabolism for the day. And just about any series of bodyweight exercises will do that. You might even want to start out by climbing up and down your stairs for two minutes. Or you might design your own two minute drill with your favourite exercises. If

MONDAY	TUESDAY	WEDNESDAY	THURSDAY	FRIDAY	SATURDAY	SUNDAY
Two-Minute Drill	Two-Minute Drill	Two-Minute Drill	Two-Minute Drill	Two-Minute Drill	Two-Minute Drill	Two-Minute Drill
Bodyweight 100	**Cardio Intervals** *Beginner* 5 min walk 15 min run/walk (total 20 min) *Intermediate* 30 min run	**Bodyweight 100**	**Cardio Intervals** *Beginner* 5 min walk 15 min run/walk (total 20 min) *Intermediate* 30 min run	**Bodyweight 100**	**Cardio Intervals** *Beginner* 5 min walk 20 min run/walk 5 min walk (total 30 min) *Intermediate* 30 min run	

you're recovering from an injury, for example, you might want to customise this morning routine to focus on simple exercises to take the stress from the problem area. The point is to do what works for you. For two minutes every morning.

What About The Rest Of The Week?

In order to make a real dent on your waistline in just one week you're going to need to work out for more than two minutes a day (sorry!) but actually, not that much more. You need just half an hour of targeted exercise each day to sear away pounds of fat, fast.

The table at the top of this page shows how the rest of Week One pans out. You'll do three resistance workouts and three cardio workouts on alternate days. The resistance workouts are known as the Bodyweight 100 and are explained in full in the next chapter. As the name suggests they require only your bodyweight, so, just like the Two Minute Drill, can be done anywhere... no excuses!

The cardio workouts are based around the concept of interval training. To start with you can set your intervals naturally, as outlined above, by slowing down when you get tired. In later weeks you will time your intervals for faster fat burning (see page 110).

GET READY! TURN FOR THE EXERCISES IN THE ALL-IMPORTANT TWO-MINUTE DRILL

BURN FAT IN TWO MINUTES

Complete as many reps as you can of each exercise in 15 seconds

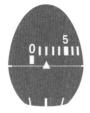

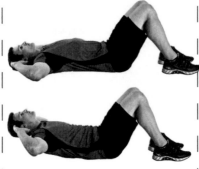

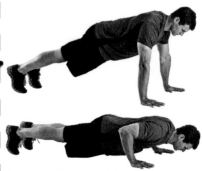

Crunches (15 seconds)

1 Lie on your back with knees bent. Keeping your neck and back straight, use your abs to lift your shoulders off the floor. Release and repeat.

Press-ups (15 seconds)

2 With body straight and hands roughly shoulder-width apart, lower yourself till your chest nearly touches the floor. Push back up and repeat.

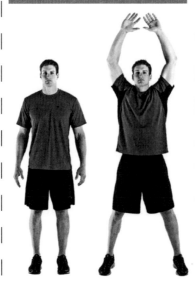

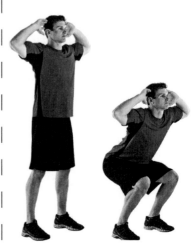

Jumping jacks (15 seconds)

5 Start with your feet hip-width apart and hands at your sides. Simultaneously raise your arms above your head and jump. Repeat.

Prisoner squats (15 seconds)

6 Stand with your chest out and elbows back. Sit back and bend your knees to lower your body. Push yourself back up and repeat.

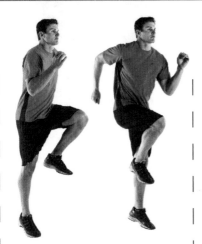

High knees (15 seconds)

3 Keeping your upper body straight, start running on the spot. Keep your knees high and swing your opposite hand for a smoother rhythm.

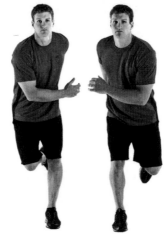

Side-to-side hops (15 seconds)

4 Starting with feet together, push off with your right foot to hop onto your left. Land on your left foot and follow with your right, then hop back.

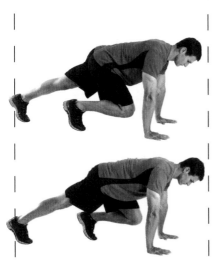

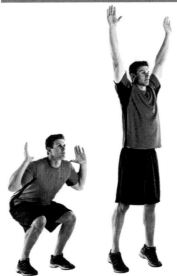

Mountain climbers (15 seconds)

7 Start in a press-up position with your shoulders directly over your hands. Bring your right knee to your chest. Extend back and repeat quickly.

Bodyweight thrusters (15 seconds)

8 Keeping your back straight, bend at the knees into a squat, then drive your legs straight while extending your arms above your head. Repeat.

CASE STUDY

Accountant **Adam Hall**, from Croydon, traded in a lardy life for winning ways and a stunning new girlfriend

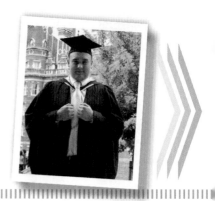

"I LIVED ON THE WORST CARBS"

A big reason many people become fat is denial. They put their expanding waistlines and plummeting fitness levels down to the ageing process rather than an unhealthy lifestyle, Adam is a case in point. "I thought being overweight was fine because I played American Football," he says, "but I was kidding myself. I was picking up injuries due to my lack of fitness, and felt low. When you're 23st, running isn't easy. Gridiron was the only cardio I did, but it's a stop-start game and I never elevated my heart rate. I couldn't run for five minutes on a treadmill."

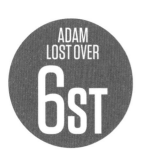

ADAM LOST OVER
6ST

Adam's unhealthy lifestyle even included weight lifting in the gym – another reason why it took him a while to wake up to his situation. "The only weights I did were infrequent bench presses and pec flys to work my chest for football. I had no idea I could be making huge inroads into my weight by working the correct muscles."

When it got to the point where he was watching more football than he was playing, Adam finally decided to take action.

BACK IN THE GAME

"Now I do three cardio sessions a week where I get my heart rate into a challenging zone. Keeping the fat off and fitness up," says Adam. "I also learnt that legs 'eat' calories, as they're your largest muscles, so I factored in leg presses and curls to build them – and their appetite – up."

"Training your legs with barbell squats creates a surge in growth hormones which help boost muscle mass," says John Foy, of The Gym Group (thegymgroup.com).

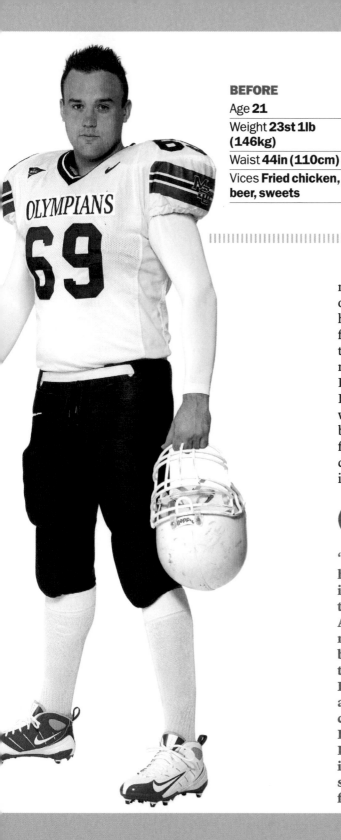

BEFORE

Age **21**

Weight **23st 1lb (146kg)**

Waist **44in (110cm)**

Vices **Fried chicken, beer, sweets**

AFTER

Age **22**

Weight **16st 10lb (105kg)**

Waist **34in (85cm)**

Victories **Confidence, new girlfriend, medals**

Adam also transformed his nutrition. "In the past I lived off the worst types of carbs," he says. "I'd get energy bursts from things like crisps, but once they faded I ate more to keep myself going. In the evenings, I ate sugary comfort food. Now I eat my big meals early, starting with a fibre and protein-based breakfast, which stops me feeling hungry later. I've also discovered crab meat: it's low in calories and high in protein."

👍 RESULT

"Now I'm fitter, faster and happier. And my 40-yard dash is down to 5.3 seconds – among the fastest on my team," says Adam "I have a wonderful new girlfriend. She knew me before I went to university as the big, quiet one. But when I saw her out after I'd dropped all the weight, I was more confident, and we got talking. I also completed the BUPA London 10K for Diabetes UK in 52 minutes – not bad for someone who couldn't run for five minutes a year ago..."

PART
TWO

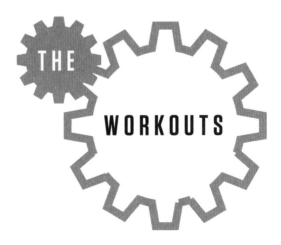

THE

WORKOUTS

5

BURN FAT WITH THE
BODYWEIGHT
WORKOUTS

**AN EASY FOUR-WEEK PLAN.
NO GYM REQUIRED**

THE FAT BURNER'S BIBLE ISN'T JUST READER-TESTED. *Men's Health* staff have also incorporated the tenets of it into their lives – and proved it really works. The pages of *Men's Health* have chronicled dozens of staff challenges and the results were published for public scrutiny. Over the years editors have burnt away literally hundreds of pounds of fat, and stacked on similar amounts of muscle. Every one of the staffers who stepped up to each challenge had demanding desk jobs on Britain's best-selling men's magazine, which put serious pressure on their free time. But they all proved that, if you have the right know-how, and a bit of discipline, it is possible to achieve your fitness goals in whatever time you have available. The workout that follows is the distilled essence a decade's worth of fat-burning knowledge.

IF YOU TAKE JUST ONE THING AWAY FROM THIS BOOK it should be this: the fastest way to burn fat is through a combination of sensible eating, cardio <u>and</u> strength training. If any one of these three pillars is not in place, your fat burning could stall. And what's the most often neglected of these three? Strength training. It's an easy trap to fall into. After all, we're constantly told that cardio workouts burn fat. Workout machines at the gym even have 'calories burned' read-outs on them so you'll never forget this – you don't get that on a dumbbell. But the less muscle you have the slower your metabolism needs to work and the fewer calories you will burn, even when you are resting. So, to really ignite your fat-burning furnace you need to do some resistance training. That's why we've developed the easiest strength building workout ever. You are going to love the Bodyweight series of workouts. Why are we so sure? Because the workouts are designed to address everything you don't like about exercise. Here's a few reasons why the Bodyweight 100 series is such a great workout and so easy to fit around your life...

❋ It's Very Quick

You've got work and volunteer commitments, home duties, friends, and family, all making demands on your time. You don't have the luxury to spend hours in a gym like an underwear model. And that's fine. Join the club. But you can carve out 20-30 minutes three or four times a week if you put your mind to it, right?

❋ You Don't Need A Gym Pass

Your nearest gym may be too far away. Too expensive. Too full of grunting muscleheads and bad music. Maybe you feel a bit intimidated because of extra weight that you may be carrying around. No problem. We're not going there.

❋ You Don't Need A Home Gym

You might not own any workout equipment but a pair of trainers. That's fine, too. For the Bodyweight 100 you won't need too much more. No expensive rowing machines or cable crossover stations. All you need is a pull-up bar, a Swiss ball and, well, you.

✴ You Don't Even Need Weights

Dumbbells have their place and you may someday want to give them a try (more on that later). But you don't have to use them to become leaner, fitter, and stronger.

✴ It's Easy To Stick To

You've tried exercise before and have always fallen off the wagon. Don't beat yourself up. We've all done that. Polls show that 50 percent of people drop out within six months. But we've got some tricks to keep you going.

✴ You'll Never Get Bored

If you feel like exercise is boring, it's probably because you're doing the same routine over and over, and you don't have a workout partner or some sort of motivational support system in place. Our plan is flexible and fun, it changes quickly to keep your interest, and it grows along with your muscles so there are always new ways to challenge your body.

These points should help to allay most of the commonly held fears people have about exercise regimes. They should help you to realise that it is possible to stick with a fitness plan, even if you have failed in the past. The programme on the following pages is flexible enough to suit anyone who wants to lose weight, whether you've just got out of shape in recent years, or have never managed to control your weight and have decided it's time to do something about it.

Stick with this programme and you'll start to see and feel results within just seven days. Once you are through the first week look on the following three weeks as your time to really master the workouts. That's the crucial period. Once you are through the first month the workouts will in *The Fat Burner's Bible* will start to become an ordinary part of your schedule – a natural part of your new lifestyle. And you will start to feel in total control of your weight and your body. Now, get ready for the Bodyweight 100.

Don't cancel outdoor running in winter. Training for just one minute at 4°C can boost your fat burning by activating brown fat, which helps to burn up regular fat reserves, found scientists at the University of Gothenburg.

WEEK 1 THE BODYWEIGHT 100 WORKOUT

Pound for pound, gymnasts are perhaps the strongest athletes in the world. And most of them rarely, if ever, lift weights. They are proof that you don't have to pump iron or use high-tech machines at the gym to build a strong and lean physique. Using the weight of your body alone is enough resistance to give yourself an exceptional workout. Bodyweight moves, after all, are the most natural of exercises and the least likely to cause injury.

Craig Ballantyne, a certified strength and conditioning specialist, longtime *Men's Health* contributor, and owner of Turbulencetraining.com, has developed the Bodyweight 100 programme. He designed it using years of knowledge and research into the best workouts for building muscle and burning fat.

The number refers to the total repetitions you end up doing in each circuit, as the weeks progress this number will increase. Week One will see you mastering the Bodyweight 100, in Week Two you'll progress to 200 exercises. These moves will prepare your muscles for the next phase of the resistance workout, Weeks Three and Four, which involve more challenging supersets.

The Bodyweight 100 is very quick, but also an extremely effective fat-burning tool. Start the session by warming up your muscles with a few minutes of star jumps or running-on-the-spot. Then do the following six moves (listed, left and described fully on the next three pages) rapidly with no rest in between exercises. Rest for two minutes after you complete this circuit, then repeat the six exercises in the same order. If you feel you can push yourself through a third circuit, rest for another two minutes, then go for it. Every extra rep you do counts. The speed and variety of each session will help you and finish with a fantastic sense of achievement and some fat well and truly burned.

EXERCISE	REPS/TIME
PRISONER SQUAT	20 REPS
PRESS-UP	20 REPS
JUMP	20 REPS
CHIN-UP	20 REPS
FORWARD LUNGE	20 REPS
PRESS-UP (CLOSE GRIP)	20 REPS
REST	2 MINS

PRISONER SQUAT

Stand with your hands behind your ears, your chest out, your elbows back, and your feet hip-width apart (A). Sit back at your hips and bend your knees to lower your body as far as you can without losing the natural arch of your spine (B). Squeeze your glutes and push yourself back to the start. That's one rep, you need to do 19 more in the Bodyweight 100.

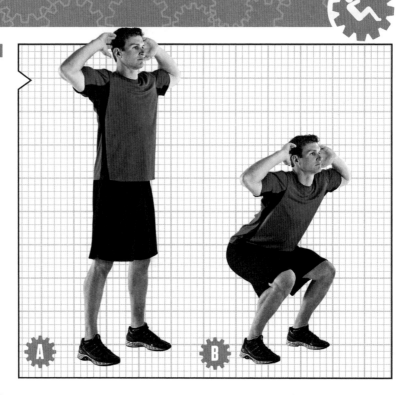

PRESS-UP

Get into the press-up position with your back and legs straight and your hands shoulder-width apart. Brace your abs and keep your body rigid (A). Now lower yourself until your chest is as close to the floor as you can get it (B). Push yourself back up until your arms are extended. If you find a full press-up too hard (and over 20 reps a lot of people do) then perform this move with your knees on the floor throughout.

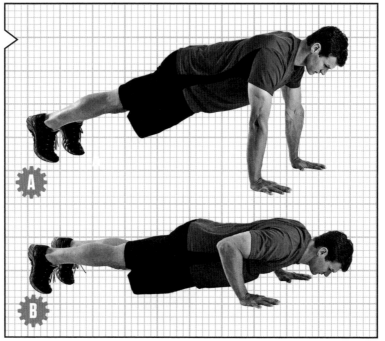

JUMP

Not quite as simple as just jumping up and down this one, but it's not far off. Master the technique to get the most out of every leap. Stand with your feet slightly more than hip-width apart. Swing your arms back as you dip down at the hips and knees (**A**). Drive your arms forward and up as you jump explosively off the floor (**B**). Immediately dip down and repeat. After 20 you'll feel the burn. But don't stop yet…

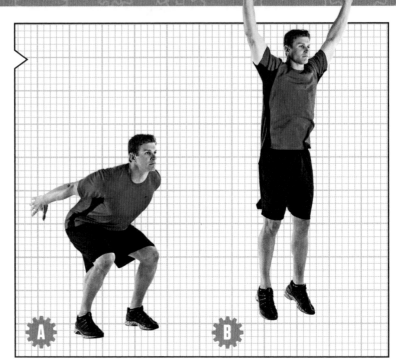

CHIN-UP

You'll need a bar for this one (try Exercise Bar, £12.98, amazon. co.uk). Hang from it as shown (**A**). Pull your chin up over the bar (**B**) then lower. This is really tough, especially over 20 reps. But don't skip it. If it's too hard, do 'negatives': start by standing on a chair at the top of the move and then take your feet off and lower yourself down slowly and repeat. For more on mastering chin-ups, turn the page.

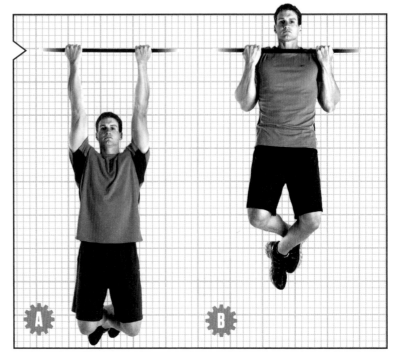

LUNGE

Don't stop! You're nearly there. And, after all those chin-ups, this one is a bit of a breather. From a standing position (A), take a large step forward with one leg. When your front thigh is parallel to the floor, keep your back knee off the floor and hold for 1 second (B). Then return to the starting position and repeat with your other leg. That's one rep. For the Bodyweight 100 you'll need 20.

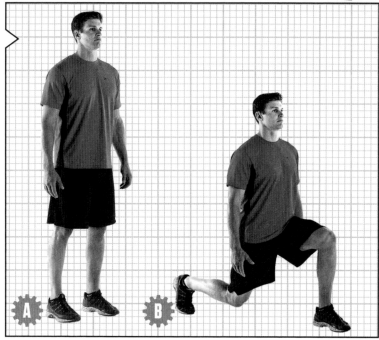

PRESS-UP
(CLOSE GRIP)

A variation on a classic. Assume the standard press-up position, but place your hands closer together, leaving about 4in (10cm) of space between your thumbs (A). Keeping your elbows tucked in against your sides, lower yourself until your chest nears the floor (B), then push yourself up. Again, if it's too difficult to complete 20 reps, do the same move with your knees on the floor.

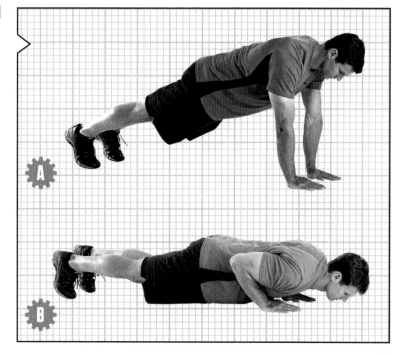

CONQUER THE
CLASSIC PULL-UP
'NEGATIVES' MAKE THIS TOUGH EXERCISE EASIER

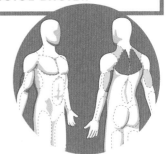

We avoid pull-ups and chin-ups for one reason: they're hard. And if you're carrying even a little extra weight, you might find them nearly impossible. That's a shame, because you'd be missing out on the best way to work the biggest muscle group in your upper body: your latissimus dorsi (as shown, right) But here's a strategy for mastering the pull-up that works...

1 LEARN THE TECHNIQUE

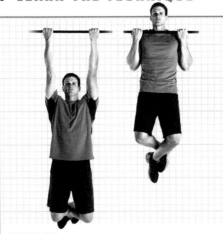

CHIN-UP

Grab the pull-up bar with a shoulder-width, underhand grip. Cross your legs and pull yourself up until your chin crosses the bar. This is a little easier than a pull-up, so good practice.

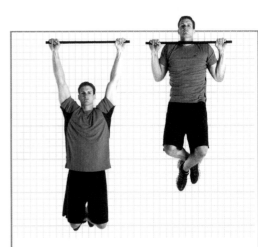

PULL-UP

The same as a chin-up but with an overhand grip. Because your biceps can't help the pull-up is harder. An easier version is to use a palms-facing (close) grip but you'll need a bar that allows this.

2 TEST YOUR LIMIT

First, determine how many pull-ups you can do. Hang from a pull-up bar using an overhand grip that's just beyond shoulder-width apart, your arms completely straight. Cross your feet behind you. Without moving your lower body, pull yourself as high as you can; your chin should rise above the bar. Pause momentarily, then lower your body until your arms are straight, and repeat. Record your total, then find the pull-up routine on this page that corresponds to your best effort. Do it twice a week, resting at least two days between sessions. After four weeks, retest yourself. Depending on your score, either advance or repeat the same routine for another four weeks. Mastering the pull-up isn't easy.

3 BECOME A PULL-UP MASTER

IF YOU CAN DO 0-1...

...improve with 'negatives'
Do only the lowering portion of the exercise. It will help you build strength for full pull-ups.

To perform a 'negative' place a bench or chair under a pull-up bar and use it to boost your body so your chin is above the bar.

Then lower your body slowly. Once your arms are straight, boost yourself up and repeat. Rest for 60 seconds after each set. Now follow the workout schedule below, using this method of 'negatives' and the time indicated for each one.

WEEK	EXERCISE	SETS	REPS	TIME
1	**Chin-up**	3	5-6	5-6sec
2	**Close-grip pull-up**	3	5-6	5-6sec
3	**Close-grip pull-up**	3	5-6	5-6sec
4	**Pull-up**	3	5-6	5-6sec

IF YOU CAN DO 2-4...

...improve with more sets
The first 1 or 2 repetitions in a set are when the most muscle fibres fire. By doing several sets of 1 or 2 repetitions, you'll activate more total fibres, increasing strength quickly. Take the number of pull-ups you can complete and half it. That's how many reps you'll do in each set. If your best effort is 3, round down to 1. Follow the workout routine below. As you can see, after two weeks, you'll increase the repetitions you are doing in each set.

WEEK	SETS	REPS	REST
1	8	**50% of best effort**	90sec
2	8	**50% of best effort**	90sec
3	8	**Best effort**	90sec
4	8	**Best effort**	90sec

IF YOU CAN DO 5-7...

...improve with more reps
To improve endurance, focus on doing more reps than normal – regardless of the number of sets it takes. So you'll shoot for 30 repetitions – even if that means you drop down to sets of 3, 2, or 1.

Perform as many pull-ups as you can, then rest for 60 seconds. Repeat as many times as needed to do 30 reps. Each workout, try to reach your goal in fewer sets. You can do 30 in one go? You are officially a pull-up master.

WEEK 2 THE BODYWEIGHT 200 WORKOUT

This week we're adding five new bodyweight exercises to the workout and increasing the total number of repetitions to 200. Also, we're throwing a new toy into the mix – a stability ball, also known as a Swiss ball.

Stability balls should really be called instability balls, because that's the secret to how they work. Supporting yourself with the ball creates instability, which forces you to use more muscles to help you balance while exercising on it. That equals better and faster results. In a recent study professor of physical therapy Dr Rafael Escamilla, and his colleagues at California State University at Sacramento, hooked electrodes to the torsos of 18 people to measure muscle stimulation while some of them exercised on a Swiss ball and others exercised without the ball. They found that ball crunches on the ball recruited twice the number of muscle fibres activated by traditional crunches or yoga/Pilates–inspired workouts. Another study in New Zealand found that press-ups using a Swiss ball trained arms 30 percent harder than regular press-ups did. "The ball forces your triceps to stabilise your elbow and shoulder joints, which results in the recruitment of more muscle fibres," according to lead investigator Dr Paul Marshal.

After warming up, do the Bodyweight 200. This includes all the exercises you learned for the Bodyweight 100 (flick back for descriptions) interspersed with the new moves you'll find described in full over the next few pages in this section. Note the changes in repetitions from Week One, especially when going back to '100' moves. If you are spent after the 200 reps, stop. If you can bang out another circuit after a five-minute rest, go for it.

EXERCISE	REPS/TIME
PRISONER SQUAT	30 REPS
PRESS-UP	30 REPS
JUMP	10 REPS
LEG CURL	10 REPS
JACKKNIFE	10 REPS
STEP-UP	20 REPS
PULL-UP	5 REPS
FORWARD LUNGE	30 REPS
PRESS-UP (CLOSE-GRIP)	20 REPS
INVERTED ROW	15 REPS
PRISONER SQUAT	15 REPS
CHIN-UP	5 REPS
REST	5 MINS

HAVE A BALL

HOW TO BUY THE RIGHT SWISS BALL

It's important to buy the right size Swiss ball. If you use one that is too small your core won't be activated properly and you'll tend to lean forward during exercises. Too big and it will be too unstable, which could be dangerous, particularly if you're lifting weights. You can tell if you are using the right one by sitting on the ball with your knees bent and your feet on the floor. If the ball is the correct size, your legs will form 90-degree angle. If you're buying online and can't test it, use the chart below to ensure you get the right size. For a good-quality Swiss ball with a pump you should expect to pay between £20 and £30. Try Studio Pro balls available at fitness-mad.com or Reebok Gymballs (escapefitness. com). They're made with burst-resistant, latex-free vinyl, which will deflate slowly and safely if it happens to be punctured.

Tip If your exercises start feeling too easy, increase the amount of air in the ball. The more inflated it is, the less stable it is, which means a more challenging workout.

Height	Swiss Ball Size
4ft 11in – 5ft 5in	55cm
5ft 5in – 6ft	65cm
6ft and taller	75cm

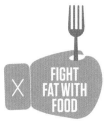

FIGHT FAT WITH FOOD

Eat bread with seeds in. It might be higher in calories per slice, but the extra fat and fibre will keep you feeling fuller for longer.

97

JACKKNIFE

This one needs a Swiss ball – see the previous page for a few handy tips on buying one. First, get into a press-up position with the tops of your feet resting on the ball, your body forming a line from toes to shoulders (**A**). Keep your back straight as you contract your abs and roll the ball toward you (**B**). Return to the starting position. Do 10 reps, then move on to the next exercise without a rest.

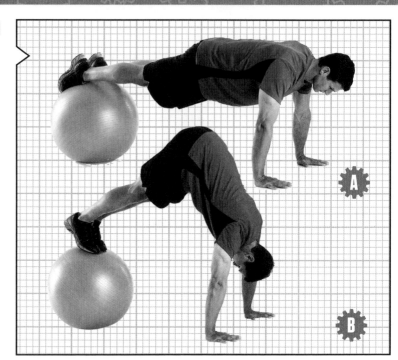

PULL-UP

Hang at arm's length from a bar with your hands shoulder-width apart in an overhand grip (**A**). Pull your chin over the bar and then lower back down (**B**). Keep your legs crossed throughout to aid balance and ensure you don't swing. These are tough, so just do 'negatives' (as described on page 94) if you can't do five. It takes time and persistence to master pull-ups, so don't get disheartened.

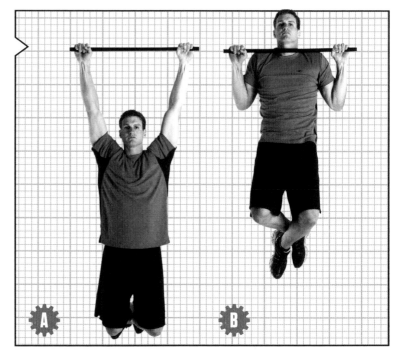

LEG CURL

This will give your legs and core a good workout. Lie on the floor with your calves on a Swiss ball and your arms at your sides. Squeeze your glutes to raise your hips off the floor so your body is in a straight line (A). Bend your legs to roll the ball towards you (B). Pause then straighten your legs to roll the ball back out. That's one rep. You need to do nine more in the Bodyweight 200.

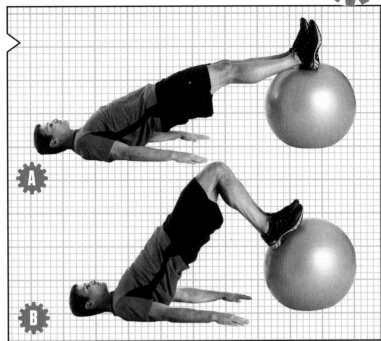

STEP-UP

Keep your blood pumping. Place your right foot on a step or bench (A) and push down through your heel to lift your left leg up until the thigh is parallel to the floor (B). Pause with your knee in the air briefly and then return to the start position. Finish all reps with one leg before switching legs and repeating. This will build muscle in you legs while giving you a cardio workout at the same time.

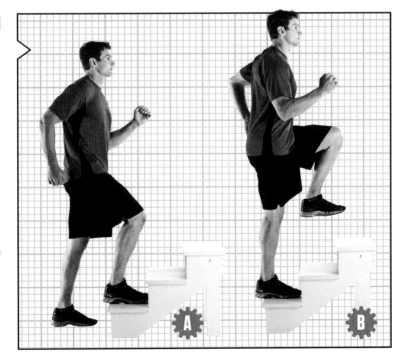

WEEK 3 **BODYWEIGHT 200 x2**

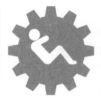

Complete the Bodyweight 200 twice, with 5 minutes of rest between circuits. Too hard? Do another week of the Bodyweight 200. Too easy? Then try the Bodyweight 200, plus the 100 exercises, with no rest between. It's your call.

WEEKS 4-6 **BODYWEIGHT SUPERSETS**

You can keep doing these Bodyweight workouts for months, mixing up the exercises to suit your mood and keep your muscles guessing – but if you're ready for the next challenge, and even greater levels of fat burning, change things up for the next two weeks by doing Bodweight Supersets.

A superset is nothing more than a workout technique that pairs two different exercises back-to-back without rest. Supersets are designed to save time and burn fat by multitasking your muscles. For example, you might work your chest and back in one superset and your legs and shoulders in another. By stressing your muscles in a short time period, you increase the rate at which your body breaks down and rebuilds protein, and this uptick in your metabolism can last for hours after your workout.

The supersets in Workout A (described in more detail over the next three pages) are listed to the left. You need to do each superset three times, resting a minute between each and five minutes before moving onto a new pair. Try doing Workout A on Monday and Friday and Workout B (consisting of another three supersets) on Wednesday. Then, the following week change them around so you're doing Workout A on Wednesday.

WORKOUT A

SUPERSET 1

SHOULDER PRESS-UP	10 reps
STEP-UP	12 reps

SUPERSET 2

SINGLE-LEG GOOD MORNING	8 reps
SWISS BALL MOUNTAIN CLIMB	20 reps

SUPERSET 3

INVERTED ROW	12 reps
WIDE-GRIP PRESS-UP	20 reps

WORKOUT A SUPERSET 1

Perform these two exercises back-to-back, with no rest in between. Rest for one minute before repeating Superset 1 twice more. Then rest for five minutes and move to Superset 2.

SHOULDER PRESS-UP
(10 reps)

Get ready for your first superset. Place your feet on a bench, step or chair and your hands on the floor. Pike your hips in the air, so that your upper body is as vertical as possible (A). Slowly lower your head to the floor (B). Pause, and push with your shoulders and triceps back to the starting position.

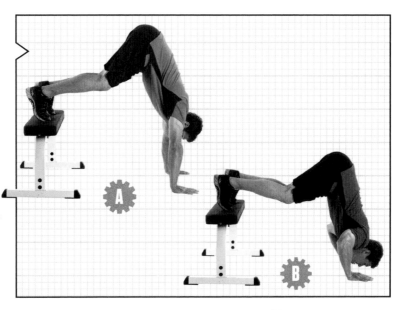

STEP-UP
(12 reps per leg)

Place one foot on a step (A) and push down through your heel to lift your other leg up until the thigh is parallel to the floor (B). Return to the starting position and finish all the repetitions with one leg before repeating the exercise with your other leg. To make the exercise more difficult, place your foot on the second step.

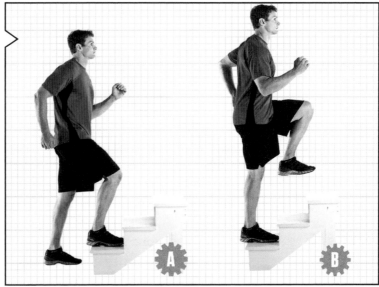

WORKOUT A SUPERSET 2

Perform these two exercises back-to-back, with no rest in between. Rest for one minute before repeating the superset two more times. Rest five minutes before moving to Superset 3.

GOOD MORNING
(8 reps per leg)

Stand with your hands beside your head (A). Raise one foot and extend it behind you. Contract your glutes, brace your abs, and keep your spine naturally arched. Lower your torso until it's parallel to the floor (B). Slowly return to the starting position. These are tough, do them slowly for 8 reps per leg.

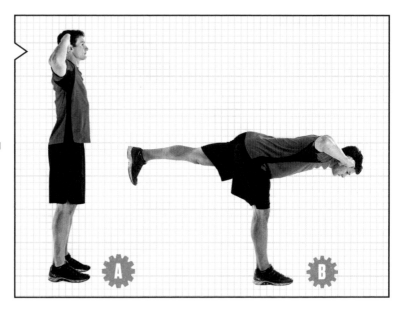

MOUNTAIN CLIMB
(20 reps)

Assume the press-up position, but place your hands on a Swiss ball, fingers pointing forward (A). Brace your abs and straighten your legs behind you. Lift one foot off the floor and bring your knee toward your chest (B). Straighten your leg back out and then bring the other knee up. That's one rep.

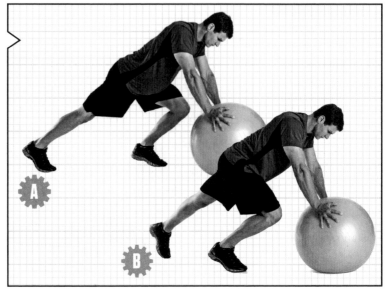

102

WORKOUT A SUPERSET 3

Perform these two exercises back-to-back, with no rest in between. Rest for one minute before repeating the superset two more times.

INVERTED ROW
(12 reps)

Set your chin-up bar in a doorway at about 3 feet from the floor or use a barbell and rack as shown. Lie under the bar and grab it with your hands shoulder-width apart (A). Keeping your body straight, pull your chest to the bar using your back muscles (B). Slowly lower yourself back to the starting position.

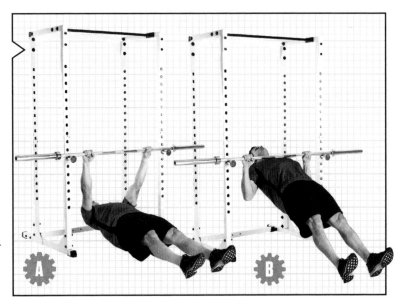

WIDE-GRIP PRESS-UP
(20 reps)

Do this as you would a standard press-up, but place your hands further apart (A). Lower slowly and focus on keeping perfect form (B). This will force more muscles to work by controlling your weight, rather than dropping suddenly. Keep up the good work – this superset is hard. Perfect for calorie burning.

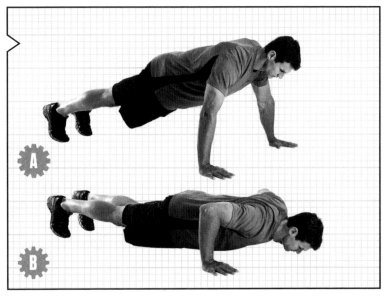

WEEKS 4-6 BODYWEIGHT SUPERSETS CONT...

This is the second part of your superset plan. Remember, you need to alternate your resistance workouts with cardio days. So if you're doing these supersets on Monday, you should do cardio intervals on Tuesday, more supersets on Wednesday, cardio on Thursday and so on (you can take Sunday off). There's more on cardio later in this chapter. It's also a good idea, when working out at this intensity, to mix up your resistance training so that you don't strain your muscles. That's why we've split these supersets into two – giving you the variety you need to ensure that you can keep on working out at maximum efficiency.

Supersets are an advanced form of resistance training, so don't get disheartened if you feel unable to progress to these workouts in Week Four. Stick with the Bodyweight 100 and these will be waiting for you when you are ready. We include them simply as the next stage. If you can do them in Week Four, great. If not, don't worry.

To help you to get the most out of your supersets, we've designed them to use compound and combination moves – exercises that work multiple muscle groups across multiple joints rather than focusing on just one muscle. By pairing noncompeting muscle groups such as your shoulders and your legs, you'll be able to push yourself even harder. Your back and deltoids will be able to rest while your hams, glutes, and calves work during the leg exercises. You'll be able to jump into your next set that much quicker, saving time. As ever, the list of exercises you need to complete in this workout is listed to the left, and then explained in greater detail over the next few pages. Good luck. And remember, the harder you push yourself the more fat you'll burn.

WORKOUT B

SUPERSET 1

PRISONER SQUAT	15 reps
WALKING PRESS-UP	8 reps

SUPERSET 2

SPLIT SQUAT	12 reps
INVERTED ROW	12 reps

SUPERSET 3

SWISS-BALL ROTATION	12 reps
WIDE-GRIP PRESS-UP	20 reps

SUPERSET 4

SPIDER-MAN PRESS-UP	12 reps
ONE-LEG HIP EXTENSION	20 reps

WORKOUT B SUPERSET 1

Perform these two exercises back-to-back, with no rest in between. Rest for one minute before repeating the superset two more times, then move on to Superset 2.

PRISONER SQUAT

(15 reps)

Stand with your hands behind your head so that your fingertips brush your ears (A). Keep your chest out and your elbows back. Sit back at your hips and bend your knees to lower your body as far as you can without losing the natural arch of your spine (B). Then push yourself back to the starting position.

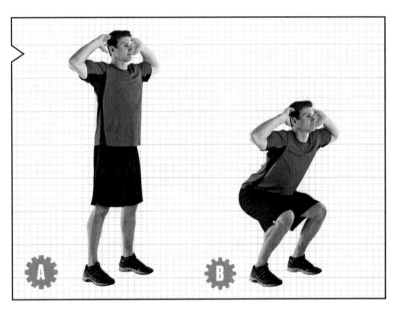

WALKING PRESS-UP

(8 reps per side)

In a press-up position put your left hand in front of your left shoulder (A). Slowly lower until your chest is an inch off the ground (B). Return to the start. Switch hand positions by 'walking' one step forward (C). Do another rep then 'walk' forward again (D). Repeat till you've done 8 per side.

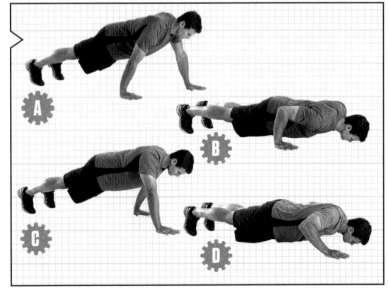

WORKOUT B SUPERSET 2

Perform these two exercises back-to-back, with no rest in between. Rest for one minute before repeating the superset two more times, then move on to Superset 3.

SPLIT SQUAT
(12 reps per side)

Stand with one foot 2-3ft in front of the other, each in line with its corresponding leg. Place the front foot on a 6in step (A). Keep your upper body erect as you descend until the top of your front thigh is parallel to the ground (B). Pause, then slowly press back up to the starting position.

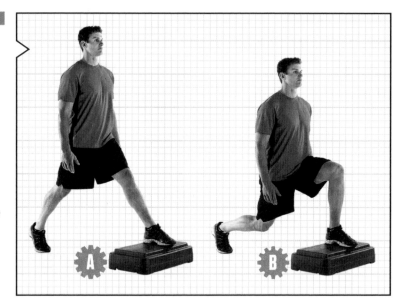

INVERTED ROW
(12 reps)

Lie face-up underneath a bar with your heels on the floor and grab the bar with your hands a little more than shoulder-width apart (A). Keeping your body in a straight line, pull your chest to the bar concentrating on using your back muscles (B). Lower yourself until your arms are straight.

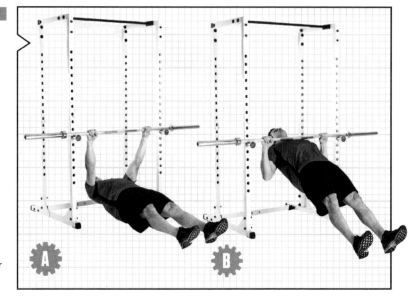

WORKOUT B SUPERSET 3

Perform these two exercises back-to-back, with no rest in between. Rest for one minute before repeating the superset two more times, then move on to Superset 4.

SWISS BALL ROTATION

(6 reps per side)

Brace your abs. Put your forearms on a bench or chair and your shins on a Swiss ball. Keep your legs straight and your back flat (A). Pull the ball forward and sideways, rolling it toward your chest (B). Pause, and return the ball to the start. Alternate until you've completed 6 reps per side.

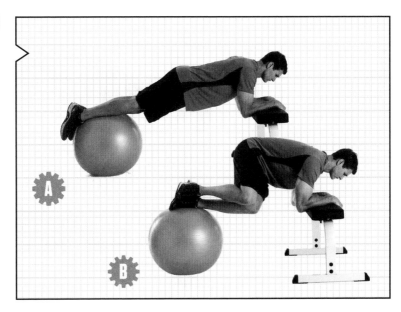

SWISS-BALL LEG CURL

(12 reps)

Lie on the floor with your heels resting on a Swiss ball. Squeeze your glutes to raise your hips off the floor so your body forms a straight line from shoulders to heels (A). Pause, then bend your legs to roll the ball towards you (B). Straighten your legs to roll the ball back to the starting position.

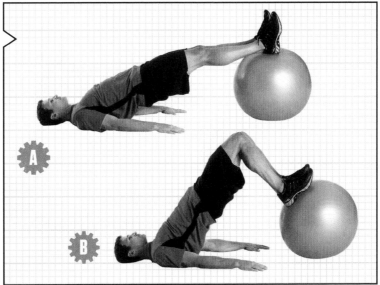

WORKOUT A SUPERSET 3

Perform these two exercises back-to-back, with no rest in between. Rest for one minute before repeating the superset two more times.

SPIDER-MAN PRESS-UP

(8 reps per side)

Assume the classic press-up position, toes on the floor, hands shoulder-width apart (A). Keeping your abs braced and your body straight, bend your elbows. As you go down, bring your right knee to your right elbow (B). Straighten your leg as you push yourself back to the starting position. Alternate legs.

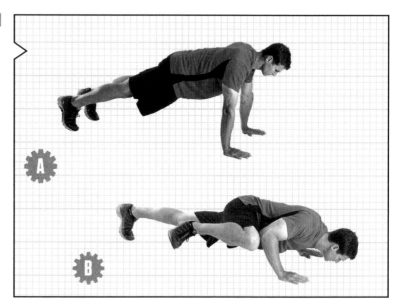

ONE-LEG HIP EXTENSION

(15 reps per side)

Lie on your back with one of your knees bent and that foot flat on the floor (A). Brace your abs while you straighten your left leg and lift it off the floor by raising your hips (B). Then slowly lower until they are nearly at the start position, but don't let your hips touch the floor. Do 15 reps then change to the other leg.

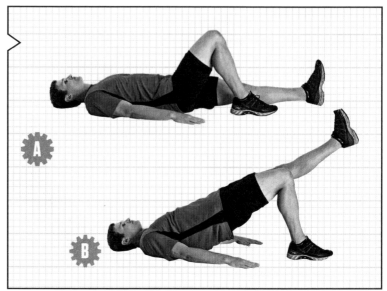

FITNESS APPS

Make cardio easy with a little handheld help

NIKE+GPS
iPhone, £1.49

This great app tracks your runs and shows them on a map. It also records your pace and tells you when you break a speed or distance record.Track your total distance and average pace, as well as sharing them on Facebook and Twitter.

SMARTRUNNER
Samsung Bada, free

Calorie, speed and distance counter (using the phone's GPS), covering 14 different sporting activities, from hiking to cycling. When you're burning fat it's great motivation to track calories. And it's difficult to do in the field without an app like this.

ADIDAS MiCOACH
iPhone & BlackBerry, free

Personalised 12-minute training sessions from top fitness coaches. "Following a varied programme means you're more likely to adhere to it – and see quicker weight loss," says personal trainer Richard Scarlett.

FITOCRACY
iPhone, Free

For computer game enthusiasts, this one is a no-brainer. Fitocracy helps motivate you to work out by giving you experience points, badges and achievements. Plus you advance to different 'levels' depending on the exercise you do.

DROIDFIT
Android, free

A set of 300 animated exercises to help you shed pounds. It also lets you record your progress. "Using proper form can help you lift more weight, which in turn helps you lose those unwanted extra pounds of fat, says weights coach Joshua Tapp.

FITNESSBUILDER
iPhone, £40 subscription

A visual way to look at workouts, with videos, pictures and calculators. This app is a complete workout and fitness solution – although very pricey. The illustrations are clear and the videos are well made, and it's a good way to keep fit for beginners.

ZOMBIES, RUN!
iPhone, £5.49

This imaginative and well-made running companion is really an interactive audiobook, set in a post-apocolyptic version of your local area. The story is delivered straight into your headphones as you exercise. This zombie-themed app gets you running for your life.

ENDOMONDO
All platforms, free

Endomondo supports a huge online community and lots of different sports including football, skiing and even dancing. Typing in your postcode will bring up local running and cycling routes. A quality app for tracking workouts and sharing them with your friends.

ADVANCED CARDIO INTERVAL WORKOUTS

WHILE THE BODYWEIGHT 100 SERIES and the superset workouts will get your heart pumping, we recommend adding interval training on the days in between your strength workouts.

As we said earlier, intervals are short bursts of high-intensity work interspersed with recovery periods of easier effort. You can do intervals with just about any type of exercise – cycling, running, rowing, swimming, skipping or exercising on an elliptical trainer or a stairclimber.

Long, slow runs are not great for burning calories. Recent studies show exercising at a higher intensity for a short period of time burns many more calories than long aerobic sessions do. Sprints fry more fat than distance running does – and a lot quicker. Canadian researchers found that high-intensity intervals were nine times more effective than endurance training at eliminating body fat. What's more, the higher the intensity of your interval workout, the longer your body will continue to burn fat and calories after you are finished exercising. This is known as afterburn, and it's the same benefit you get from rigorous weight lifting. The bottom line is this: if you want to incinerate fat, you have to increase the intensity of your workouts whenever possible.

On the next page are some examples of simple running interval workouts. You should perform them on the days in between your strength workouts or, if you feel ambitious, right after a resistance workout. Before each workout, warm up for five minutes by exercising at an easy pace (this should be about 30 percent of your full effort). After you're finished, cool down for five minutes in the same manner.

If you prefer to do your cardio outdoors then running over undulating hills or even a long, steady climb can create a natural interval workout. Just run as fast as you can for as long as you can up the hill, then jog slowly or walk until you've caught your breath, and then repeat. Simple.

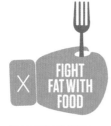

FIGHT FAT WITH FOOD

Researchers at the University of Zagreb have found that fish and yoghurt boost your metabolism. Their iodine encourages your thyroid gland to release hormones that signal your body to burn fat.

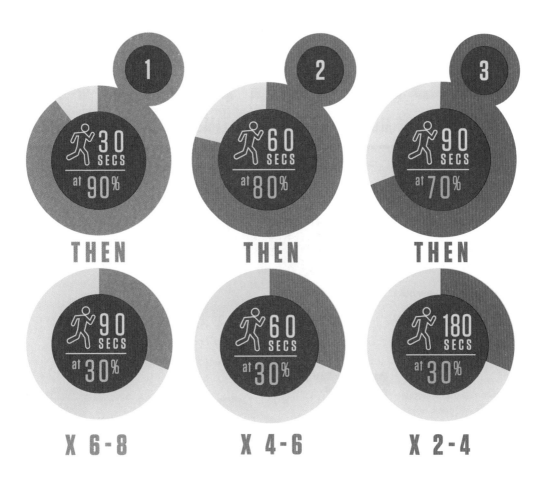

1

🏃 30 SECS
at 90%

THEN

🏃 90 SECS
at 30%

X 6-8

2

🏃 60 SECS
at 80%

THEN

🏃 60 SECS
at 30%

X 4-6

3

🏃 90 SECS
at 70%

THEN

🏃 180 SECS
at 30%

X 2-4

If you prefer exercising on a bike, it's often easiest to do intervals in the gym, as sprinting down busy roads (or even country lanes) can be a little dangerous on two wheels. Here's a good bike workout: after a warm-up, go all out for 30 seconds, then recover for 30 seconds. Do 10 cycles of that sequence, then pedal hard for 60 seconds followed by 60 seconds of recovery pedalling for five sets. Finally, pedal for another five minutes, this time changing gears to increase or decrease resistance at 15-30 second intervals.

THE WORLD'S BEST
BODY STRETCH

A FIVE-STAGE MOVE THAT WILL SAVE TIME AND BEAT SORENESS

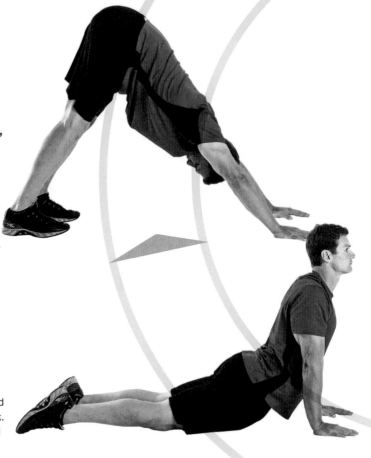

Finally, slowly lift your butt, straightening your legs while pointing the top of your head to the floor. Your body should form an upside-down V. Your feet should be flat on the floor. Try to keep your heels down. You'll feel the stretch in your hamstrings and back. Hold for 30 seconds.

Next, raise your head up while lowering your hips toward the floor and arching your back. Your head should point toward the ceiling. Feel the stretch? Contract your shoulder blades to open up your chest. Hold for 30 seconds.

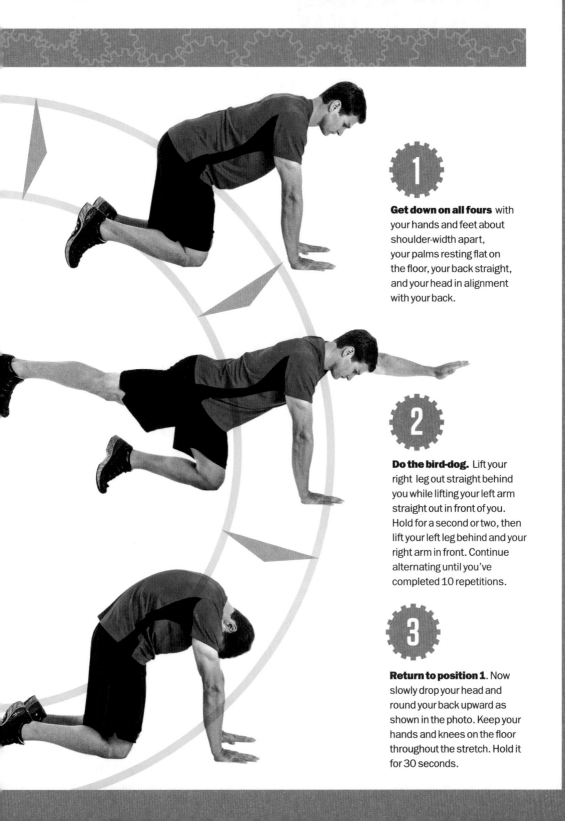

1

Get down on all fours with your hands and feet about shoulder-width apart, your palms resting flat on the floor, your back straight, and your head in alignment with your back.

2

Do the bird-dog. Lift your right leg out straight behind you while lifting your left arm straight out in front of you. Hold for a second or two, then lift your left leg behind and your right arm in front. Continue alternating until you've completed 10 repetitions.

3

Return to position 1. Now slowly drop your head and round your back upward as shown in the photo. Keep your hands and knees on the floor throughout the stretch. Hold it for 30 seconds.

CASE STUDY

Knee problems meant **Daniel Hawkes**, from Surrey, struggled to run off his 21st. So he got on his bike. Follow in his slipstream...

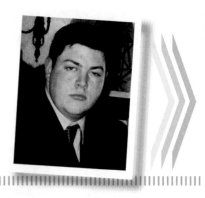

"I HAD TO BATTLE WITH AN INJURY"

Daniel piled on fat as a student thanks to excessive snacking and huge portion sizes, by his mid twenties he had busted the 20st mark and felt depressed about his weight, as he felt that changing it was out of his control. "Then I read about one of the Fat-burners of the Month in *Men's Health*. This guy had been my size and now looked great," says Daniel. "I tore out the tips and used them for inspiration."

"I ditched the television in my kitchen and entertained myself by cooking recipes from scratch every night." Take a leaf out of Daniel's cook book and listen to music as you prepare meals: a study of at-home weight loss published in the *Annals of Behavioral Medicine* found dieters with fewer TVs in their home lost around 10% more body weight and then kept it off.

THE RIGHT KIT

"I got a heart-rate monitor, which gave structure to my regime," says Daniel. "It's great for targeted fat-burning." To exercise efficiently – improving stamina and burning fat – aim for the magic window between 65% and 75% of your maximum heart rate. You can judge this roughly as running at the speed at which you are still just able to hold a short conversation. But using a heart-rate monitor makes it much easier to hit exactly the right level.

"A misaligned kneecap meant I had to find low-impact cardio solutions. So I started commuting by bike (13 miles each way) three times a week, which worked off the fat, without making my knee

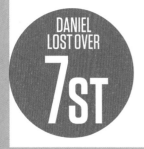

DANIEL LOST OVER

7ST

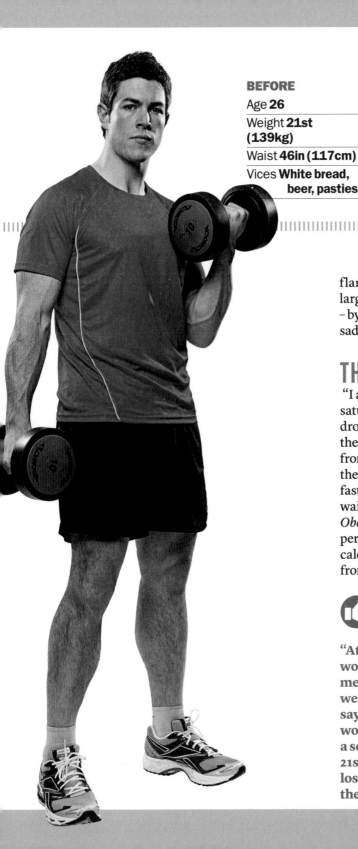

BEFORE	AFTER
Age **26**	Age **27**
Weight **21st (139kg)**	Weight **14st 12lb (94kg)**
Waist **46in (117cm)**	Waist **36in (91cm)**
Vices **White bread, beer, pasties**	Victories **"Normal" clothes and marriage**

flare up." Challenge your largest muscles – your glutes – by regularly standing up in the saddle when you get on your bike.

THINK DRINK

"I also got rid of foods full of saturated fats, which helped me drop to 18st 7lb. Then I ditched the soft drinks and cut out sugar from tea and coffee." Drinking the wrong beverages is the fastest way to blow out your waistline. A study in the journal *Obesity* showed the average person takes in 21% of their calories – around 460 a day – from drinks alone.

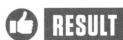 **RESULT**

"At 15st I met Abby. She was wonderful at encouraging me to stick to my regime and we got married last April," says Daniel. "I know she wouldn't have given me a second look when I was 21st, but thanks to my weight-loss plan I'm now married to the woman of my dreams."

6

THE
DUMBBELL
WORKOUTS

> ## LIFTING WEIGHTS CAN BUILD MORE
> ## MUSCLE AND BURN MORE FAT

DID YOU KNOW THAT AFTER YOU HIT 30, you will lose some muscle mass with each passing year? Unfair, isn't it? It means after you waive goodbye to your twenties, your body will probably never be as Speedo-friendly again, but more importantly, it means that with less muscle, your metabolism is slower and it will be easier for fat to accumulate, especially around your middle. The same goes for you, if you're over 30. And you know how dangerous abdominal fat can be.

AS WE LEARNED EARLIER, how much your metabolism stays fired up after your workout is directly related to the amount of muscle tissue you engage. So, our new dumbbell workout targets the largest muscle groups in the body – the chest, back, shoulders and legs. A University of Wisconsin study found that when volunteers performed a full-body workout involving just three big-muscle exercises – the bench press, power clean, and squat – their metabolisms were elevated for 39 hours afterwards. In addition, researchers discovered that these lifters also burned a greater percentage of their calories from fat during this time, compared with people who didn't do a total-body, big-muscle workout. Many of the exercises in this programme go one step further: they combine two lifts in one exercise to work multiple large muscle groups, to deliver an even better metabolism charge while saving you workout time.

Here are some more reasons to add weights to your workout—and reasons to make them dumbbells:

Weights Push Your Muscles Harder

Once your body gets used to doing the exercises in the Bodyweight programme, your muscles will stop growing, and this is not because you are doing anything wrong. It will happen to everyone. Seasoned weight lifters call this phenomenon plateauing. You reach a level at which your exercise isn't as effective. But by adding weights to your training, your muscles will stay challenged and continue to grow. A higher muscle density gives you a higher basal metabolic rate – meaning you burn more calories, even when not exercising. It's basically a win-win situation.

Weights Strengthen Your Whole Body

Studies have shown that lifting weights can reduce your blood pressure, make your heart pump blood more efficiently, and reduce the amount of artery-clogging cholesterol in your blood. Other studies indicate that the act of stressing your skeleton with weights can even make your bones stronger and less prone to fracture.

THE WEIGH TO GO

HIGH-TECH SCALES TRACK FAT BURNING <u>AND</u> MUSCLE BUILDING

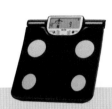

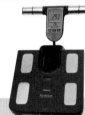

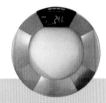

Tanita BC 601, £160

Muscle weighs more than fat, so it's important to get a set of scales that measures both – if you're burning fat and building muscle your weight might not drop as fast as you expect. These top-end scales give information on your entire body, plus specifics on dangerous visceral fat.

Available at Tanita.co.uk

Omron BF511, £50

Features foot sensors and hand controls to give accurate body-fat readings. These scales also highlight visceral fat and, crucially, measure upper body fat separately, which is often a key problem area for men. Ideal for men who are after targeted, precision weight loss.

Available at Boots.com

Tanita BC 570, £50

These scales measure body fat, muscle-mass and metabolism. The 'athlete's mode' gives modified readings for more muscular frames. You might not be at 'athlete' level yet, but even building a small amount of muscle could skew your weight readings, so it's worth investing in good scales.

Available at JohnLewis.co.uk

Dumbbells Prevent Injury

Because dumbbells allow a greater range of motion, you can work out in three dimensions rather than the static up-and-down or side-to-side motions to which barbells and machines limit you. This helps you engage smaller muscle fibres that are extremely important in supporting your joints and larger muscles. The stronger your supporting muscles are the less injury prone you will be. If you use a bar instead of dumbbells, your wrists get locked into a position that can press on nerves and cause pain, much like repetitive strain injury. Dumbbells, on the other hand, let you adjust your wrists to help take the pressure off during certain lifts.

USE DUMBBELLS TO REACH THE NEXT LEVEL

 Before you get started, there's a law of muscle physics to learn that will help you get quicker results from your lifting: the law of elastic energy. When you lower the weight during any exercise, you build up elastic energy in your muscles. Just like in a coiled spring, that elasticity allows you to bounce back to the starting position, reducing the work your muscles have to do. It's unintended cheating, but if you eliminate this cheating bounce, you'll force your body to recruit more muscle fibers for a better workout. Pause for about 3 seconds in the down position of an exercise: that's the amount of time it takes to discharge all the elastic energy of a muscle.

There's another benefit to this strategy: lowering a weight with control will force your muscles to work harder, stimulating more growth and burning more calories. So you can increase size and strength of muscles by pausing on the down phase of a lift. Keep these points in mind as you do the following dumbbell exercises. Alternate Workouts A and B over 3 lifting days each week. Do 2 sets of 8-12 repetitions each. That'll take you 15-20 minutes.

DUMBBELL WORKOUT A	REPS/TIME
BULGARIAN SPLIT SQUAT	8-12 REPS PER LEG
DUMBBELL STEP-UP	8-12 REPS PER LEG
DUMBBELL BENCH PRESS	8-12 REPS
SEATED DUMBBELL SHOULDER PRESS	8-12 REPS
BICEP CURL	8-12 REPS
DUMBBELL SINGLE-ARM ROW	8-12 REPS PER ARM
CRUNCH	1 SET TO FAILURE

WORKOUT A

(Mondays and Fridays)

BULGARIAN SPLIT SQUAT

Grab a pair of dumbbells and stand with your back 2-3 feet (60-90cm) from a bench. Place your right foot behind you on the bench so that your foot rests on it. Hold the dumbbells at arm's length at your sides (A). Keeping your torso upright, lower your body until your left knee is bent 90 degrees and your right knee nearly touches the floor (B). Pause, then push yourself back to the starting position as quickly as you can.

That's one rep. Do 8-12 repetitions, then place your left foot on the bench and repeat the exercise this time with your left foot behind you on the bench.

Master this move with light weights first before progressing to heavier dumbbells. Remember you always need to challenge your muscles in order for them to grow and this move will hit some of the biggest muscles in your body.

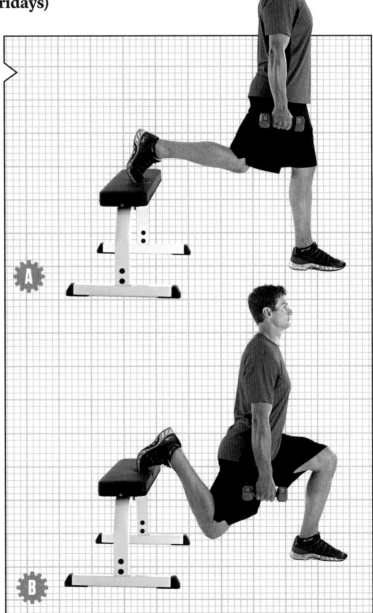

121

DUMBBELL STEP-UP

Grab a pair of dumbbells and hold them at your sides. Stand facing a bench or a sturdy chair or bench, and place your left foot on it (A). Push your body up until your left leg is straight and you're standing on one leg on the bench (B). Lower your body until your right foot touches the floor. That's 1 rep. Do 8 to 12 reps with your left leg, then repeat the exercise with your right leg.

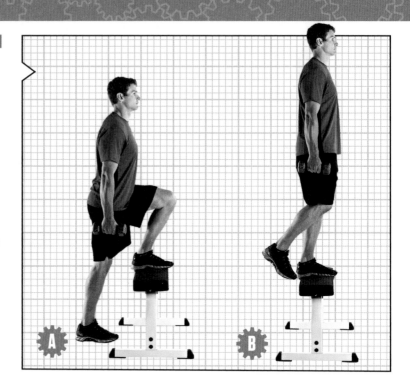

BENCH PRESS

This classic move is still unrivalled for building your chest. Lie on a flat bench holding a pair of dumbbells at arm's length above your chest, with your back in a normal arch (A). Lower the dumbbells slowly towards the sides of your chest (B) (stop when your elbows are at bench level or just a little lower), pause, then push them back up to the starting position. Do 8-12 reps.

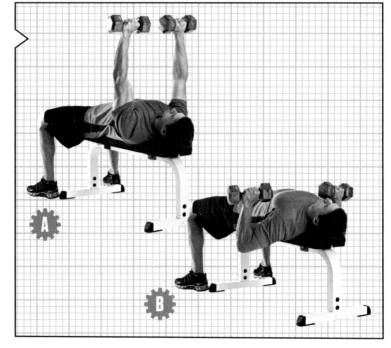

SHOULDER PRESS

Sit on an exercise bench holding a pair of dumbbells. Lift them up just above your shoulders (A), and with your feet flat on the floor, press the weights up until your arms are straight up above your head (B). Pause, slowly lower, and then repeat. If you have any mild pain in your shoulders you can do this move with a neutral grip, palms facing each other, to ease strain on your joints.

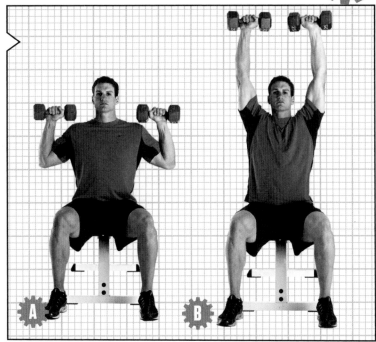

BICEP CURL

Stand holding a pair of dumbbells at your sides (A). Keeping your upper arms perfectly still, curl the weights up, rotating your forearms so the move finishes with you holding the weights in an underhand grip in front of your shoulders (B). Pause, lower, and repeat. Keep your muscles engaged throughout the motion for maximum efficiency. Perform 8-12 reps.

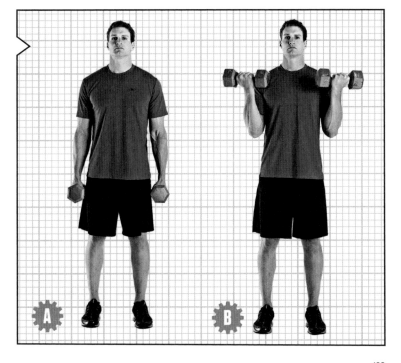

SINGLE-ARM ROW

Grab a dumbbell in your right hand and place your left hand and left knee on a flat bench. Keep your back flat and your upper body parallel to the floor. Put your right arm straight down (**A**) and raise until your elbow is above the level of your torso (**B**). Pause, lower, and repeat. You should feel tension in your back muscles if you're doing this right. Do 8-12 reps, then repeat the with your left hand.

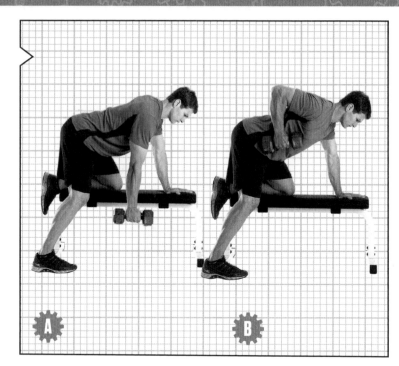

CRUNCH

Lie on your back with your knees bent and hands behind your ears (**A**). Slowly crunch up, bringing your shoulder blades off the floor (**B**). Then return to the starting position. Do as many crunches as you can. Keep your abs tight throughout the motion, pause for a moment at the top of the move. Don't lock your fingers together or pull on your neck during this move – this is an easy way to strain a muscle.

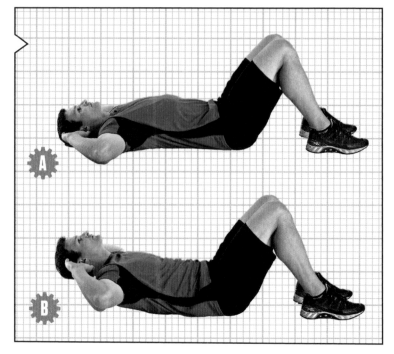

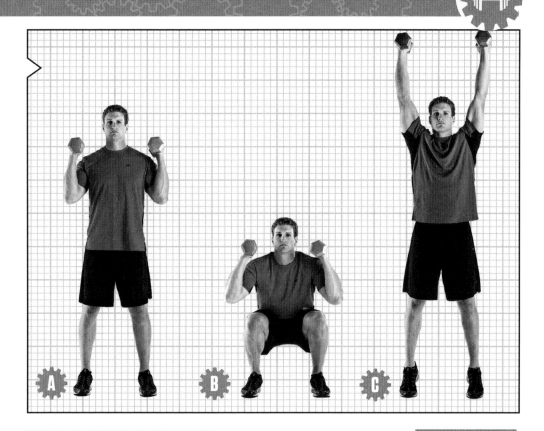

WORKOUT B

(Wednesdays)

DUMBBELL WORKOUT B	REPS/TIME
DUMBBELL THRUSTER	8-12 REPS
WALKING LUNGE	8-12 REPS
SWISS-BALL PRESS	8-12 REPS
SWISS BALL CRUNCH	1 SET TO FAILURE
CROSS PUNCH	15-20 REPS PER ARM
CORKSCREW	1 SET TO FAILURE

DUMBBELL THRUSTER

Hold a pair of dumbbells by your shoulders (A). Position your feet shoulder-width apart, then quickly lower until your thighs are parallel to the floor (B). Explode back up and push the dumbbells above your head (C). Pause, then lower the dumbbells as you squat back down and repeat.

WALKING LUNGE

Grab a pair of dumbbells and hold them at your sides (A). Stand with your feet hip-width apart. Step forward with your right leg and slowly lower your body until your right knee is bent 90 degrees and your left knee nearly touches the floor (B). Your right lower leg should be perpendicular to the floor, and your torso should remain upright.

▶ ▶ ▶

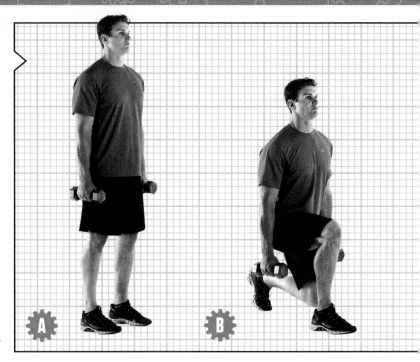

SWISS-BALL PRESS

Like a regular bench press, get yourself into position, only instead of a bench your upper back, shoulders and head are supported by the ball. Your feet on the ground as normal. Raise both dumbbells (A). Now, lower one dumbbell (B) and then drive it upward. As you're driving the dumbbell up, lower the other dumbbell (C). You need to have lowered both weights once to count as one rep

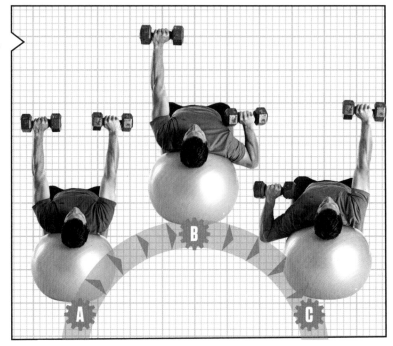

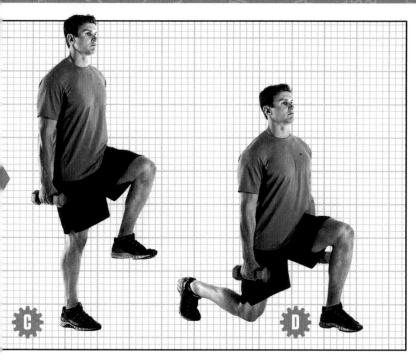

▶ ▶ ▶

Pause momentarily, then push off your right leg (C) and step forward with your left leg so that your body is in the starting position again, but a full lunge step ahead of where you began (D). (That's right, you'll be walking forward with each lunge, so give yourself some room.) Then repeat, lunging forward with your left leg. That's 1 repetition. Do 8-12, alternating legs.

SWISS-BALL CRUNCH

Sit on a Swiss ball with your feet flat on the floor, shoulder-width apart. Walk your feet forward and stop when your knees are bent at 90 degrees (A). Keep your head in line with your upper body, place your hands behind your ears and draw in your abs. Raise your chest up and slightly forward in a crunching motion (B). Pause, slowly return to the start, then repeat. Do as many as you can.

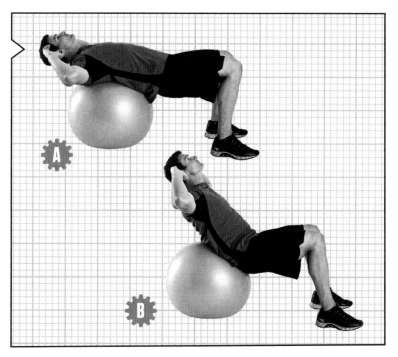

CROSS PUNCH

Stand holding a pair of light dumbbells in front of you, palms facing in (A). Punch your right fist forward and to the left across your body (B). Draw your arm back as you punch with your left fist. Perform 15 to 20 repetitions with each arm. This works your biceps and chest. Also, if you keep your core tight throughout it will be a great workout for your abs and obliques.

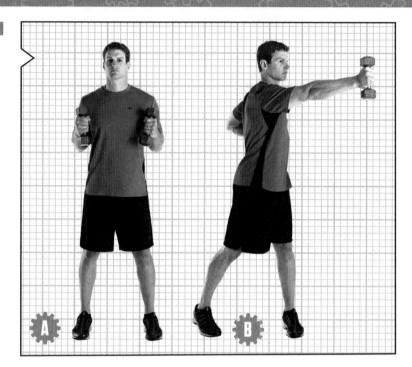

CORKSCREW

Lie on your back with your legs directly over your hips. Your knees should be slightly bent. Place your hands as shown (A). Use your lower abs to raise your hips off the floor and toward your rib cage, elevating your feet straight up. Simultaneously twist your hips to the right (B). Hold for a second, and then return to the starting position. Repeat the exercise, this time twisting to the left.

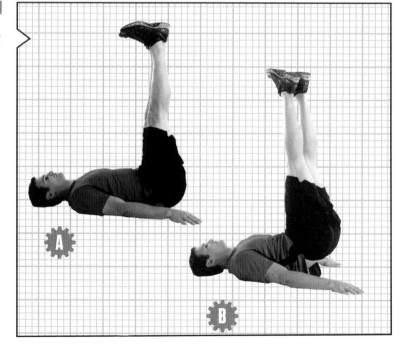

WORKOUT BOOSTERS

14 WAYS TO ENSURE YOUR REGIME IS SUPER-EFFICIENT

Over the years, we've collected some tweaks and tips from the best trainers and exercise physiologists in the business. Here's a handful of our favorites for you to work into your workouts.

1 SMILE WHEN YOU STRETCH It's hard to be tense when you are grinning. Try it. Letting all the tension out of your neck, shoulders, and arms will help you achieve a deeper, more effective stretch.

2 TRY DROP SETS Doing 5 reps or fewer per set with a weight that you can lift only five times trains your muscles to grow bigger and stronger, says Mark Peterson, an exercise and sport scientist at Arizona State University. Do 3-5 sets without rest, reducing the weight by 10-25 percent each set.

3 NEVER SKIP YOUR CRUNCHES After you bench-press, do 25 crunches on the bench. You'll be less likely to skip them than if you have to go find an exercise mat.

4 CHANGE YOUR GRIP It can help you do more repetitions. Try a set of barbell curls with a narrow grip. When you begin to fail, slide your hands out further. You'll get more out of your biceps.

5 USE YOUR LEGS FOR SHOULDER PRESSES. Just a slight dip of the knees as you start each shoulder press will help you push more weight over your head. Your legs won't help you lower the load, so your shoulders reap the rewards.

6 MOVE WEIGHT TO THE FRONT FOR SQUATS It's easier to keep your back upright – and avoid injury – if you hold the weight across your chest, not behind your neck. This position also generates more power.

7 USE A MIRROR WHEN LIFTING It's much easier to check your technique when you can see yourself. You'll build more muscle and help to prevent injury.

8 ADD A SHRUG. Instead of lowering the weight at the top of a standing shoulder press, lock your elbows, pause, and shrug as if you were trying to touch your shoulders to your ears. Your trapezius and deltoids will benefit.

9 NEVER WAIT FOR EQUIPMENT Your body is the best fitness tool you have. Next time a bench is bustling, add a set of press-ups or another bodyweight move from this book to your routine.

10 SQUEEZE YOUR KNEES Lie on your back with knees bent 90 degrees and feet flat on the floor. Place a Swiss ball between your knees. Lift your hips until only your heels, upper back and head touch the floor. Then lower. This works your hamstrings and will help to prevent groin pulls.

11 TAKE DEEPER, SLOWER STEPS when you're on on the stairclimber machine. You'll burn more calories and work your leg muscles more fully than if you take short, choppy steps.

12 GO LONG The longer your stride when running, the more effective your workout will be, according to University of Idaho researchers. They found that an extended stride length on cardio equipment can boost oxygen consumption by up to 12 percent and heart rate by 6 percent.

13 FLIP YOUR GRIP to become instantly stronger. Scientists at the National Strength and Conditioning Association's annual conference, reported that men who performed the deadlift with an alternating grip – one hand grasping the bar overhand, the other underhand – could complete two more reps than when they used the traditional grip.

14 STAGGER YOUR SQUAT STANCE To do this simply move one foot a few inches ahead of the other when you are performing squats. Do it every third workout. It will prevent your dominant leg from doing more than its fair share of the work.

CASE STUDY

Manny Prabhu smashed through his weight-loss plateau. Here's how you can emulate his phenomenal achievement

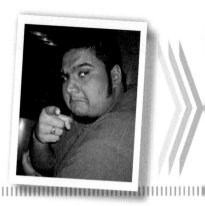

"JUNK FOOD ALMOST RUINED ME"

Manny went to college in America, but sadly the land of the burger went straight to his gut. "Although my girlfriend tried to keep me healthy, I'd gorge on fast food," he says. His girlfriend knew a thing or two about staying in shape as she was a cheerleader, but even her motivational miniskirt and pom-poms weren't enough to distract him from his love of eating.

"She put me on a diet but I went behind her back – with junk food – and we split up." Manny's body then started crying out for help: "At 17st (108kg) I started to suffer with

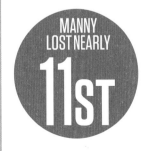

MANNY LOST NEARLY 11ST

joint pain," he says. "I decided a change of surroundings would help me best and moved back to England."

ARNIE INSPIRED

Manny got a place at Leeds University to continue his studies and there joined a gym and got chatting to a personal trainer. "He gave me the DVD *Pumping Iron*. Seeing Arnie talking about motivation and his 'one more rep' mentality inspired," says Manny. "After losing my first 1.5 stone (10kg), I had a lot more energy for studying. Compound exercises brought my weight down another 4st (25kg)." Studies show resistance work fires up your metabolism for up to 18 hours after your workout. Add squats, bench-presses and deadlifts to your routine to burn more calories than cardio alone.

MADE TO MEASURE

Once he started losing weight, Manny started to get militant about what he ate. Out went

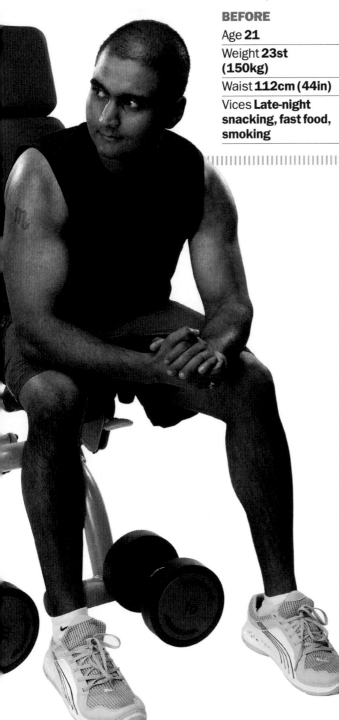

BEFORE

Age **21**

Weight **23st (150kg)**

Waist **112cm (44in)**

Vices **Late-night snacking, fast food, smoking**

AFTER

Age **23**

Weight **12st 4lb (78kg)**

Waist **86cm (34in)**

Victories **Improved health, happy and excited about life**

the junk food, in came a new, scientific approach to nutrition. "I measured out meals with scales," says Manny. "A portion of meat should be about the size of a deck of cards." See Chapter One for more tips on how to judge portion sizes when you don't have a set of scales handy.

"I reached a plateau at around 16.5 stone (105kg), so I took this as a cue to change my diet again – drinking more green tea and reducing the carbs in my evening meal. My daily calorie intake dropped down from about 2,200kcal to more like 2,000kcal."

👍 RESULT

Manny hit his target weight of 12st 4lb (78kg) in just under two years and now feels healthy and excited about the future and all it holds. He is determined that he will never go back to his old ways. "I now stick to small plates of food, snacking on nuts before bed," he says.

PART
THREE

EATING RIGHT

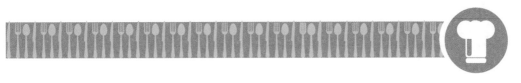

⑦

YOUR EASY
RECIPES
FOR SUCCESS

**EASY RECIPES AND SIMPLE SHOPPING LISTS
FOR REAL FOOD THAT TASTES GREAT**

EATING IS ONE OF LIFE'S SUPREME JOYS. Just think about how delightful it is to tuck into a slab of ribs slathered in barbecue sauce, or a masterfully grilled tuna steak. To crunch into a crisp garden salad drizzled with extra-virgin olive oil and balsamic vinegar. Life should be about eating that way. Eating well. And savouring every bite. You don't want to deny yourself the pleasure of eating good food. Yet most diets ask you to do just that and that has a lot to do with why those diets are destined for failure. Diets that force you to deny yourself your favourite foods are virtually impossible to follow for any length of time. Having willpower is empowering, but sacrificing can be extreme and ultimately too difficult for most. Eat well, and eat healthy.

THE *MEN'S HEALTH* PHILOSOPHY IS THIS: we strongly believe that if you make smart choices from a variety of food groups, exercise practical portion control, and break a sweat most days of the week, you can generally eat whatever you wish. We understand that you're human. You get hungry. Flavour and satisfaction are important. And when you've done a good job at whatever it is that you do, you deserve a good meal. Unless your doctor demands it, there's really no reason that you should have to stop eating steak or Chinese food, or go cold turkey on pizza. They aren't the dietary devils they've been made out to be. It's how we eat them and how much of them we eat that can cause us trouble. It's those bad choices we're making – heavy on the processed foods and sugary and calorie-laden snacks – that pile on the pounds.

On the following pages, you'll find recipes for *The Fat Burner's Bible* Recipes for Success. These are traditional favourites for breakfast, lunch, and dinner. We didn't select them because they're ultra-low in fat or carbohydrates or calories. If we did, you wouldn't eat them – because they'd taste like cat litter. We did, however, try to keep them full of all the good stuff you want when you're keeping an eye on your health, and kept the portions reasonably sized. Whenever possible, we suggest recipes that prepare one serving to help you avoid overeating.

All these meals taste good. We've tried them. And they're easy to prepare, too. That's important. Recipes with too many steps or too many ingredients and pots and pans are a complete turn-off. And Simpler is always better. We've all been there – when we're single and lazy, our dinners are all simple: hamburgers, instant white rice with a can of tuna dumped over it, microwaved ready-meals with gelatinous sauces and bits of unidentifiable meat.

Ordering takeaways online, microwave meals and fast food make it easy to avoid cooking four or five times a week. This is what we've kept in mind when choosing these recipes: things we'd like to eat, and things we frequently do. Restaurant-quality and healthy needn't be mutually exclusive, and neither should easy and tasty. These recipes are all of these things, keeping your belly off and satisfying your hunger, while being easy enough to cook after a long day's work or a hard session at the gym. We want you to impress

NUTRITION APPS

Construct a fat-burning menu with your phone

RESTAURANT NUTRITION	WEIGHT-LOSS SENSEI	THIN-CAM	DIET FITNESS DIARY
iPhone, free	**BlackBerry, £1.50**	**iPhone, £0.59**	**BlackBerry, £2.49**

RESTAURANT NUTRITION

iPhone, free

A calorie database of hundreds of British restaurants. It'll tell you how many calories that burger really has in it.

"We generally underestimate our daily calorie intake by about 25%," says sports nutritionist Yolanda Hinchcliffe of sukasport.com.

WEIGHT-LOSS SENSEI

BlackBerry, £1.50

This clever app draws on the expertise of behavioural psychologists and dieticians to draw up eating plans for you, tailored specifically to your lifestyle.

"Tracking your daily meals will flag up where there's room for improvement in your diet," says Hinchcliffe.

THIN-CAM

iPhone, £0.59

You upload photos of your meals. Experts then analyse your habits and suggest improvements.

"We forget the BLTs – bites, licks, and tastes – we take each day," says Hinchcliffe. "Each one has an average of 25 calories." This helps you to monitor your real intake.

DIET FITNESS DIARY

BlackBerry, £2.49

This helps you to record what you eat, then suggests ways of shaving off calories.

As you'll know from Chapter Two, keeping a food diary can double you weight loss. As you probably carry your phone on you at all times, this app cuts down on your chances of missing an entry.

your mates, your girlfriend, or someone else's girlfriend with your culinary prowess, without having to worry about the calorie content of each mouthful.

All of the ingredients for the recipes should be available in your local supermarket, so there's no need for trips to specialist health food shops. *The Fat Burner's Bible* is about keeping the things you love, while losing the thing you hate. Your food should be no exception to this rule. From snacks and breakfasts to lunches and dinners, these recipes are tried and tested *Men's Health* classics, so cook 'em up and tuck in.

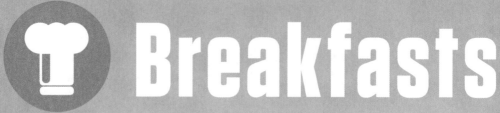

Breakfasts

BACON & EGG MUFFIN

2 large eggs

1 large pinch flaxseeds (whole)

1 wholemeal muffin, toasted

1 slice extra-lean bacon

1 slice low-fat cheddar

Cherry tomatoes

- Poach the eggs, grill the bacon and toast the muffin
- Melt the slice of cheese for 30 seconds in the microwave on full power
- Put the bacon and eggs on the muffin and top with the melted cheese
- Sprinkle with flaxseeds
- Serve with tomatoes on the side

 MAKES 1 SERVING
Per serving: 335 calories, 31g protein, 31g carbs, 10g fat (3g saturated), 5g fibre

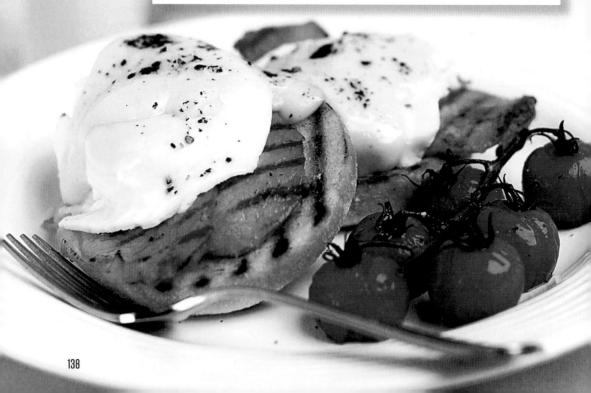

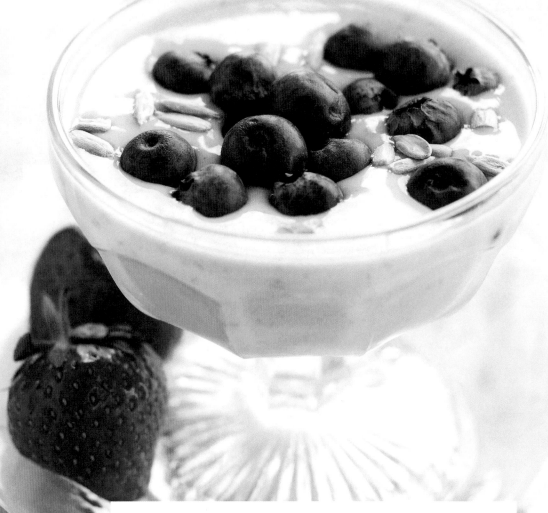

QUICK THICK YOGHURT+

250g low-fat plain yoghurt

1 handful blueberries

A few almonds

1 large handful granola (optional)

- Spoon the yoghurt into a bowl
- Stir in the blueberries, almonds, and granola (optional)

MAKES 1 SERVING

Per serving: 366 calories, 15g protein, 42g carbs, 16g fat (1g sat), 7g fibre

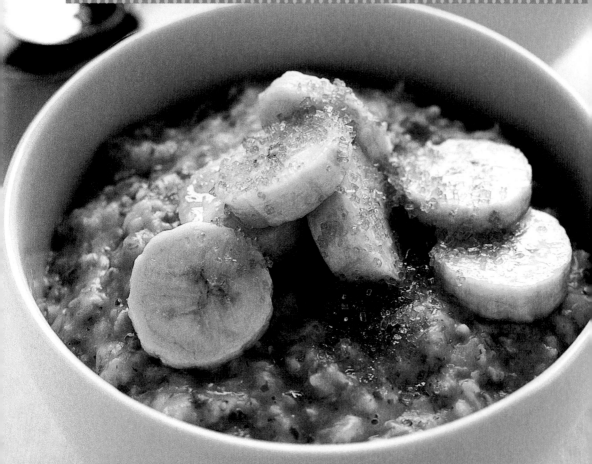

PROTEIN-POWER PORRIDGE

90g rolled oats

½ pint skimmed milk

1 scoop whey protein powder

½ banana

Sugar to taste (optional)

- Combine the oats and milk in a large microwavable bowl

- Microwave for 1 minute, stir, then microwave for another minute

- Let the porridge cool for a minute then mix in the protein powder (it's important to let it cool slightly or the protein powder can go lumpy)

- Top with banana and sprinkle with a little sugar if desired

MAKES 1 SERVING

Per serving: 585 calories, 43g protein, 80g carbs, 11g fat (4g saturated), 10g fibre

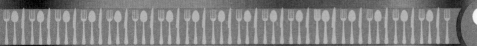

BREAKFAST SMOOTHIE

Handful of ice

Handful of chopped pineapple

A few blueberries

A few raspberries

120g low-fat yoghurt

- Grab your fruit, ice and yoghurt and throw it in a blender
- Blend until smooth
- Pour into glasses or into a Thermos flask for cool-all-day smoothies

MAKES 1 SERVING

Per serving: 252 calories, 5g protein, 68g carbs, 3g fat (0g saturated), 5g fibre

You can use any combination of fruit and yoghurt to make this a tasty way to get one of your five-a-day. Try using green tea instead of yoghurt for a fruity iced tea mix.

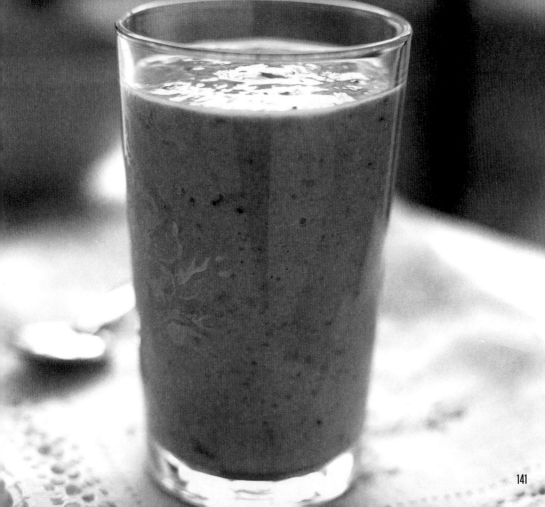

COUNTRY OMELETTE

2 spring onions, chopped

1 green chilli, chopped

1 red pepper , chopped

Olive oil

2 eggs

Splash skimmed milk

Salt and pepper

Handful grated low-fat cheddar

Baby spinach

- Fry the spring onions, chilli and pepper for a few minutes in a little oil, then transfer to a bowl

- Wipe out the pan; coat thinly with olive oil. Leave it on a medium/high heat

- Mix the eggs and milk together very briefly (you still want to see yolk, you're not making scrambled egg) with a little salt and pepper

- Fry without stirring for a minute then add the vegetables and cheese

- Fry for another 3-4 minutes until the eggs are set. If necessary tip the pan slightly so uncooked egg runs to the edges where it will cook more quickly

- Sprinkle with spinach and a little salt if desired serve

MAKES 1 SERVING

Per serving: 288 calories, 34 g protein, 13g carbs, 11 g fat (5 g saturated), 2g fibre

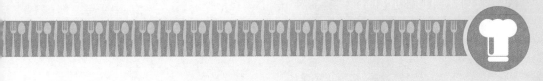

HOT BREAKFAST BURRITO

1 large wholemeal tortilla

2 large eggs,

A small handful of cheddar

1 tomato, chopped

2 tbsp salsa

- Place the tortilla on a chopping board
- Scramble the eggs
- Add the cooked eggs to the tortilla and top with the cheese, tomato and salsa. Fold
- Grill for 2 minutes to crisp up the tortilla if desired

MAKES 1 SERVING

Per serving: 419 calories, 43g protein, 28g carbs, 14 g fat (4g saturated), 2g fibre

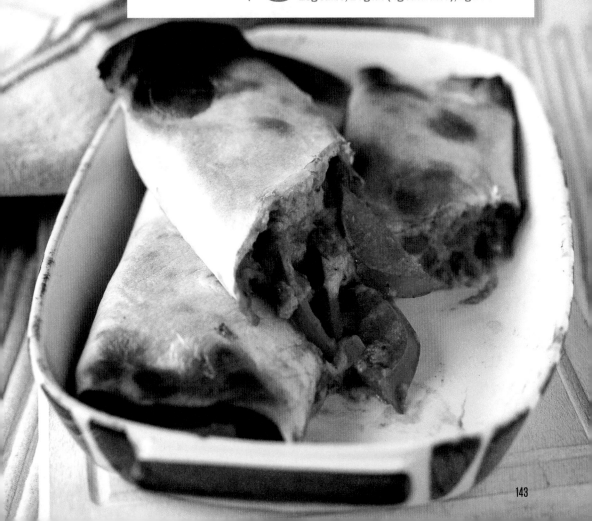

Lunches

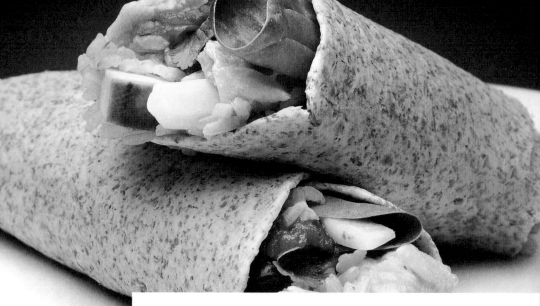

MEDITERRANEAN WRAP

1 large wholemeal tortilla

2 tbsp hummus

A few roasted red pepper strips

4 slices roast turkey breast

Baby spinach

1 avocado, chopped

Mint leaves and mango pieces (optional)

- Lay the tortilla flat on a chopping board. Spoon the hummus evenly over it
- Layer on the other ingredients
- Fold in the sides and then roll to form a wrap. Cut diagonally in half for that fancy deli look

MAKES 2 WRAPS

Per serving: 328 calories, 35g protein, 31g carbs, 7g fat (0.5g saturated), 4g fibre

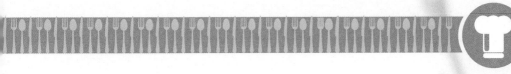

PRAWN AND PASTA SALAD

80g brown pasta

100g cooked prawns

1 avocado, chopped

A few cherry tomatoes, halved

Lettuce or other salad leaves

1 tsp olive oil

- In a medium pot of boiling water, cook the pasta for 8-10 minutes. Drain and rinse until cool

- Place the pasta, prawns, avocado, tomatoes, lettuce and olive oil in a large bowl and toss to coat

MAKES 2 SERVINGS

Per serving: 99 calories, 10g protein, 10g carbs, 3g fat (0.5g sat), 2g fibre

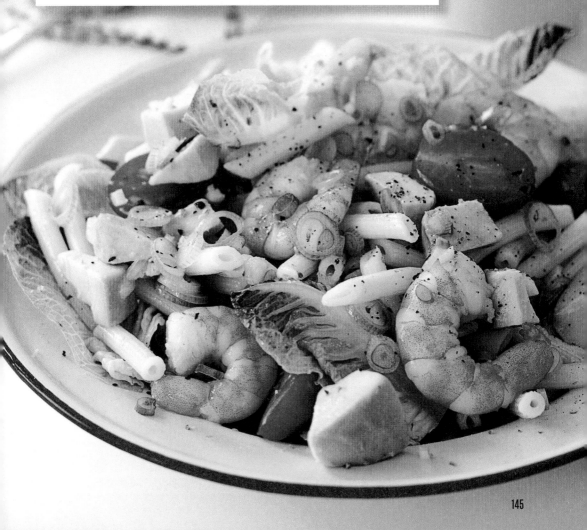

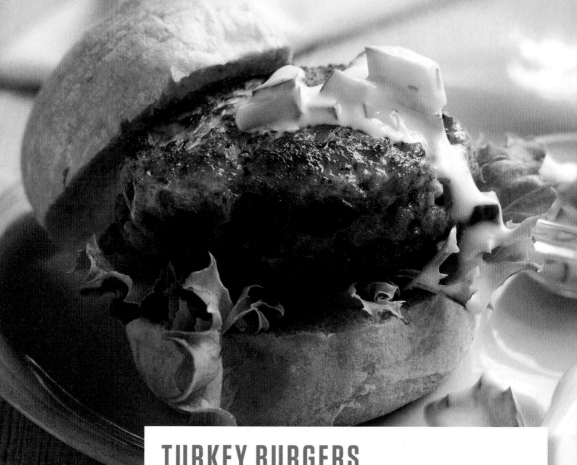

TURKEY BURGERS

250g turkey mince (use lean beef if you can't find turkey)

Salt and pepper

1 tomato, sliced

½ red onion, thinly sliced

2 wholemeal buns, toasted

Lettuce leaves

1 avocado, sliced

2 tbsp low-fat sour cream

- Compact the meat, salt and pepper into two equal patties
- Preheat a griddle pan over medium-high heat
- Cook the burgers 4-5 minutes per side, until slightly firm to the touch
- Dress each bun with tomato and red onion and lettuce
- Add the burger and top with sour cream and avocado slices

MAKES 2 SERVINGS

Per serving: 419 calories, 38g protein, 37g carbs, 21g fat (5g saturated), 3g fibre

GARDEN PIZZA

1 bag wholemeal pizza dough (£2.50, tesco.com)

2 tbsp pesto

½ head broccoli, chopped

1 red pepper, sliced

80g mushrooms, sliced

1 red onion, sliced

2 tsps olive oil

60g low-fat mozzarella cheese, thinly sliced

- Preheat the oven to 230°C/gas mark 8
- Roll out the dough as thinly as you can
- Spread the base with pesto
- Lightly fry the broccoli, peppers and mushrooms in a little olive oil
- Top the crust evenly with the cheese. Arrange the sautéed vegetables over the cheese and bake for 18-20 minutes, until the crust is baked through and crisp
- Let stand a few minutes before cutting into quarters

MAKES 4 SERVINGS

Per serving: 301 calories, 16g protein, 42g carbs, 11 g fat (3 g saturated), 7g fibre

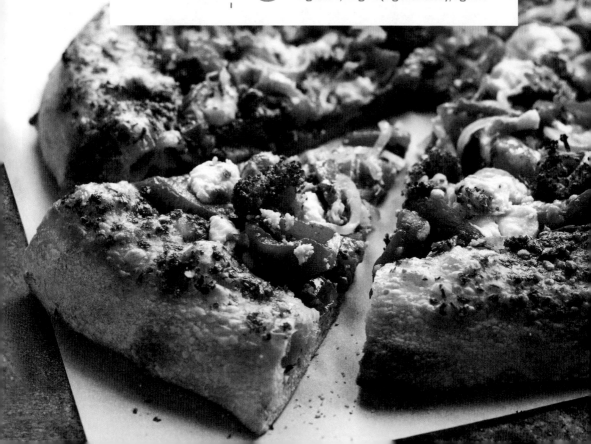

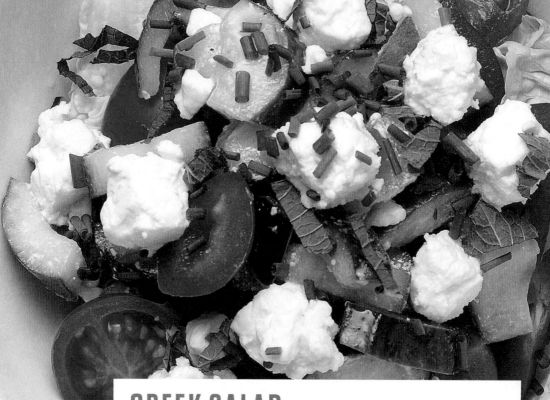

GREEK SALAD

1 head gem lettuce

½ red onion

½ cucumber

100g low-fat feta

1 medium tomato

2 tbsp lemon juice

2 tsp olive oil

A dollop fat-free yoghurt

Dried oregano

A few chives, chopped

Salt and pepper

- Chop the lettuce, onion, cucumber, tomato and feta
- Combine the ingredients in a large salad bowl
- In a jar, combine the lemon juice, oil, yoghurt and oregano; shake to mix. Add salt and pepper to taste.
- Pour over the salad. Toss well
- Top with chopped chives

MAKES 4 SERVINGS

Per serving: 48 calories, 1g protein, 6g carbs, 2g fat (0.5g saturated), 2g fibre

COLD HOT TUNA SANDWICHES

A dollop of low-fat mayonnaise

½ teaspoon wasabi paste

1 tin of tuna

8 slices wholemeal bread

Half a red onion, finely chopped

1 red pepper, sliced

1 tomato, sliced

A few lettuce leaves

- In a small bowl, mix the mayonnaise and wasabi paste together
- Fork the tuna into the bowl and combine with the mayo-wasabi mixture
- Spread equal amounts of the spicy tuna mixture on 4 slices of bread
- Top each with onion, a pepper ring, a tomato slice, a lettuce leaf and a slice of bread

MAKES 4 SERVING

Per serving: 308 calories, 22g protein, 34g carbs, 10g fat (2g saturated), 7g fibre

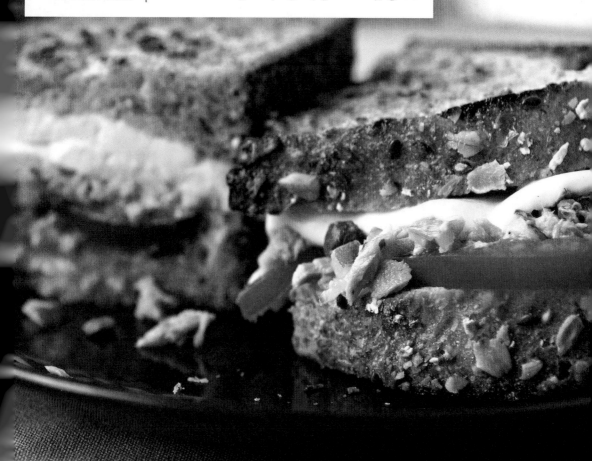

THE ULTIMATE
SALAD

QUICK, EASY AND EXTREMELY NUTRITIOUS

Salad is actually makes a brilliant meal for men. Mostly because it involves demolition. You chop and dice vegetables and tear hunks of crisp lettuce with your bare hands; and no matter how uncoordinated you are, you just can't get it wrong. If you can make a mess, you can make a salad. Stick it in a bowl and you've got a meal.

START WITH A BASE

SPINACH

This powerful green leaf is a good source of folate, which a study in the journal *Stroke* found can help to reduce your risk of stroke by as much as 20 percent, if you get some every day. It's also been linked with a 13 percent decrease in your risk of heart disease.

PINE NUTS

These are full of good fats and muscle-building protein, which will help to fill you up and stop you reaching for the bread basket. Toast them lightly in a frying pan for a few minutes before spinkling them on. This will add to the flavour by taking away any bitterness.

THEN ADD

CHEESE

Four cubes of Swiss cheese provides 476 mg of calcium and 26 international units (IU) of vitamin D. In a 20-year study, British researchers determined that men who consume more than 190 mg of calcium and 67 IU of vitamin D a day have half the risk of stroke of men who consume less.

TINNED TUNA

Tuna, one of the best sources of protein, contains 11 mg of heart-healthy niacin, which has been shown to help lower cholesterol and help your body process fat. University of Rochester researchers found niacin raises HDL cholesterol and lowers triglycerides more than statins.

BROCCOLI

You get about 300mg of potassium in a small portion. According to Mayo Clinic researchers, potassium counteracts the effects of salt by dilating blood vessels and helping to cleanse your body, thus lowering blood pressure and giving you protecting against stroke.

PEPPERS

Yellow peppers are a particularly good source vitamin C. According to a study in the *Journal of the College of Nutrition*, levels of C-reactive protein—a blood marker for inflammation linked to heart disease—can be decreased by 24% by eating 500 mg of vitamin C a day.

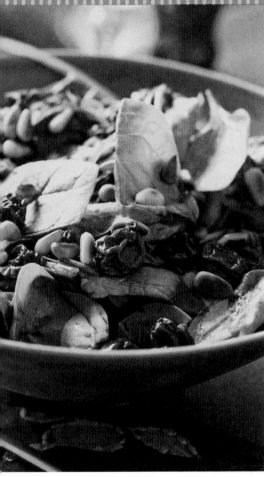

NUTRITION FACTS

Calories 618

Protein 41g

Carbs 35g

Fat 37 g (6g saturated)

Fibre 14g

Salt 0.4g

(Figures based on complete salad using all ingredients on this page)

RAISINS

These are full of healthy natural sugars: great for a pre-workout energy boost. They're also high in fibre to aid digestion and calcium to supercharge your fat-burniging. Their delicious sweetness will create an excellent balance with the savoury flavours.

DRESSING

Your best option is olive oil and balsamic vinegar. One tablespoon of oil has about 10g of monounsaturated fat, which will help to boost your testosterone levels, meaning you'll build fat-searing muscle more easily. Recent the fat will help to aid nutrient absorption.

CARROTS

Carrots are one of the richest sources of carotenoids – antioxidants that fight disease. Just 40g of carrots provides three times your RDA of vitamin A. According to a study in the journal *Thorax*, beta-carotene can slow the age-related decline of lung power.

TOMATOES

Tomatoes contain the only nutrient proven to protect against prostate cancer – lycopene. A study at Harvard University found it could reduce the risk of this disease by as much as 43 percent. They are also high in vitamins A and C and calcium and potassium.

KIDNEY BEANS

This superfood is full of disease-fighting antioxidants, plus there's 3g of fibre in every 40g serving. The American Dietetic Association, found fibre lowers cholesterol and helps normalize blood glucose and insulin levels, decreasing the risk of heart disease.

ALMONDS

One tablespoon of almonds provides 2.2g of alpha-tocopherol, a type of vitamin E, which reduces the risk of Alzheimer's, according to a National Institute on Aging study. Another study showed that people who were depressed had lower levels of alpha-tocophero.

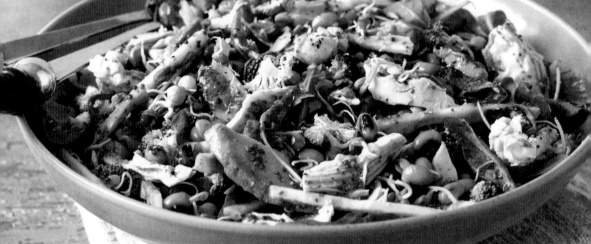

Dinners

TURKEY-AVOCADO SALAD

2 tbsp cider vinegar

1 tsp Dijon mustard

3 tsp olive oil

450g cooked turkey breast, chopped

1 packet baby spinach

4 slices cooked lean bacon, chopped

1 diced avocado

4 cherry tomatoes, halved

Ground black pepper

30g blue cheese, crumbled (optional)

- Combine 2 tbsp water, vinegar, mustard, and 2 tsp of the olive oil in a bowl, and mix well

- Put the spinach and 2 tbsp of the dressing into a large salad bowl, and toss to coat the leaves

- Arrange the turkey, bacon, avocado, tomatoes, and cheese over the spinach carefully, especially if you are entertaining. (If it's only for you, just chuck it on.)

- Drizzle on the remaining dressing, and season with black pepper to taste

MAKES 2 SERVINGS
Per serving: 288 calories, 34 g protein, 10g carbs, 14g fat (3 g saturated), 3g fibre

SUPER SIRLOIN STEAK

1 large sirloin steak

A generous splash of balsamic vinegar

Black pepper

1 clove garlic

A splash of olive oil

- Mix the vinegar, pepper, garlic, and olive oil in a large zip-top bag, reserving enough for drizzling. Drop the steak into the bag and shake to coat. Put the bag in the refrigerator for at least an hour, or overnight

- Grill the steak in a griddle pan for about 2 minutes per side for medium. Baste with the reserved marinade

- Slice and drizzle with any leftover marinade

- Serve with any steamed green veg you fancy

MAKES 1 SERVING
Per serving: 393 calories, 48 g protein, 8 g carbs, 14 g fat (6 g sat), 0 g fibre

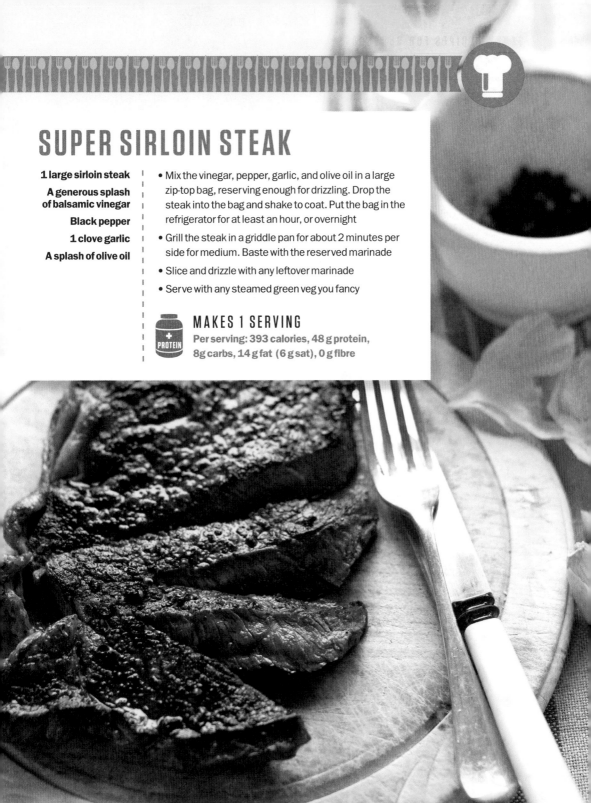

QUICK, SPICY SEA BASS

A splash of olive oil

2 sea bass fillets

1 small onion, sliced

A few stalks of asparagus

2 cloves garlic, finely chopped

1 finely chopped chilli

6 cherry tomatoes

Low-fat mayonnaise

- Heat a frying pan over medium-high heat. Add the olive oil
- Season the fish with salt and pepper. When the oil is hot, add the fillets skin-side down and cook for 3 minutes, until the skin is crispy. Remove from the pan and set aside
- Add the onion to the pan and cook for 3 minutes. Add the garlic and chilli and cook for another 3 minutes. Season with salt and pepper
- Return the fish to the pan. Cook until the flesh flakes with gentle pressure from your finger (5-7 minutes)
- Serve with cherry tomatoes, drizzled with olive oil and low-fat mayonnaise

LOW CARB

MAKES 2 SERVINGS

Per serving: 400 calories, 35g protein, 13g carbs, 19g fat (2 g saturated), 2 g fibre

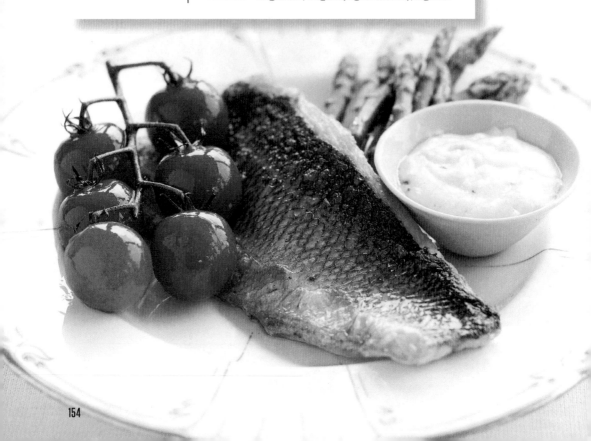

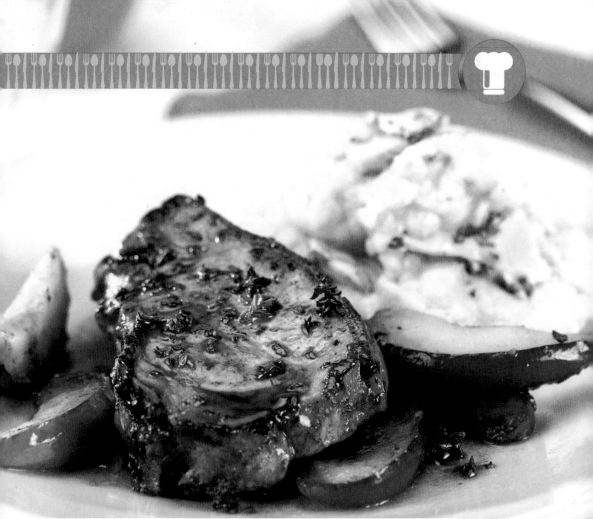

PEACHES AND PORK CHOPS

1 head cauliflower

2 pork chops

Olive oil

Fresh thyme leaves

Salt and pepper

1 tbsp Balsamic vinegar

2 firm peaches, sliced

1 knob butter

- Boil the cauliflower for 4-5 minutes
- Preheat a griddle pan on high. Brush the pork with olive oil and season with thyme, salt and pepper. Grill for 4-5 minutes on each side.
- Brush a little Balsamic on the peaches. Add to the pan and grill until soft.
- Drain the cauliflower and mash with thyme leaves and a little butter

MAKES 2 SERVINGS

Per serving: 430 calories, 38g protein, 16g carbs, 24g fat (9g saturated), 2g fibre

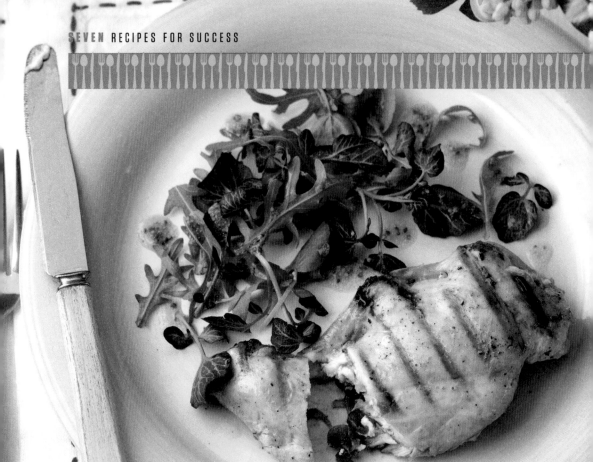

GREEK-STYLE STUFFED CHICKEN

Handful chopped sun-dried tomatoes

Handful crumbled low-fat feta cheese

Handful chopped black olives

1 clove garlic, finely chopped

1 tablespoon Balsamic vinegar

2 chicken breasts

Olive oil

Salt and pepper

Salad leaves

- Preheat the oven to 220°C/gas mark 7
- Toss together the tomatoes, feta cheese, olives, garlic and vinegar
- Rub the chicken with olive oil, salt, and pepper
- Carefully cut a slit along the thick part of each chicken breast, creating a pocket. Add enough stuffing to fill each pocket and transfer to a baking tin
- Bake for 25 minutes. Top with any remaining stuffing
- Serve with a little some mixed salad leaves dressed with a little olive oil

MAKES 2 SERVINGS

Per serving: 480 calories, 45g protein, 9g carbs, 23g fat (5g saturated), 4g fibre

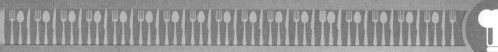

ONE-POT TURKEY CHILLI

1 onion, chopped

1 clove garlic

200g turkey mince

1 tin chopped tomatoes

½ tin kidney beans

1 tsp chilli powder

1 fresh chilli, chopped

1 small pepper, chopped

A large dollop of low-fat sour cream

- Heat some olive oil in a large pan
- Fry the onion and garlic over medium-high heat
- Add the chilli powder and fresh chilli and fry for a few minutes more to create a spicy paste
- Add the mince to the pan and break up with a wooden spoon and cook through (7-8 minutes)
- Stir in the tomatoes with their juice, kidney beans. Bring to a boil on medium-high heat
- Cover, turn down the heat to medium-low, and cook on medium for an hour – an hour and a half won't hurt.
- Serve topped with sour cream and some of the raw, chopped pepper

MAKES 6 SERVINGS

Per serving : 299 calories, 30g protein, 19g carbs, 6g fat (2.7g saturated), 8g fibre

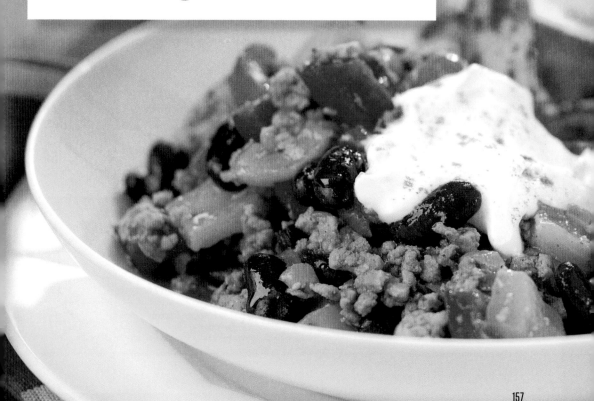

SUPER-SMART
FOOD SWAPS

CUT CALORIES WITHOUT SACRIFICING FLAVOUR

Eat This...	Not That...	Calories saved
CARBOHYDRATES		
Wholemeal muffin with blueberry fruit spread	Blueberry muffin	SAVE **270** CALS
Wholemeal pitta	Hamburger bun	**55**
½ large baked potato	Mashed potatoes	**100**
1 slice wholemeal toast topped with ½ banana and 1 teaspoon peanut butter	3cm thick slice banana bread	SAVE **260** CALS
A serving of oatmeal	A serving of granola	**125**
One portion of brown rice mixed with frozen vegetables and 1 teaspoon olive oil	A serving of white rice with 2 teaspoons butter	**65**
A serving of wholemeal spaghetti, a small handful of sliced mushrooms, a serving of marinara sauce	A serving of white spaghetti with a serving of meat sauce	SAVE **160** CALS
DRINKS		
Water with a squeeze of lemon	500ml soft drink	SAVE **180** CALS
330ml bottle of light beer	500ml can of beer	**100**
330ml latte made with fat-free milk	500ml latte made with whole milk	**120**
Large iced coffee, skimmed milk	Large iced Mocha Cookie Crumble Frappuccino	SAVE **471** CALS
½ cup juice cut ½ cup water	1 cup juice	**60**

Eat This…	Not That…	Calories saved
SNACKS		
Sliced raw vegetables	Tortilla chips with salsa	**100**
Pizza topped with sliced grilled chicken	Pizza topped with pepperoni	**100**
4 squares of dark chocolate	1 large chocolate chip cookie	**SAVE 180 CALS**
2 scoops ice cream with a handful of sliced strawberries	4 scoops ice cream on its own	**100**
A handful of unshelled pistachios	A handful of Peanut M&Ms	**90**
A bag of baked crisps	A bag of crisps	**50**
A large handful of air-popped popcorn	A handful of crisps (about 15)	**95**
A few diced strawberries with small serving fat-free vanilla yoghurt	1 large fruit-on-bottom yoghurt	**SAVE 105 CALS**
DAIRY		
1 tablespoon Parmesan cheese	4 tbsp grated Cheddar cheese	**SAVE 90 CALS**
8 tbsp reduced-fat mozzarella	8 tbsp grated whole mozzarella	**85**
8 tbsp semi-skimmed ricotta cheese	8 tbsp whole-milk ricotta cheese	**45**
3 large egg whites	2 large eggs	**SAVE 95 CALS**
PROTEIN		
200g skinless chicken breast	200g chicken breast with skin	**60**
200g filet steak	200g T-bone steak	**120**
200g turkey meatloaf	200g beef meatloaf	**SAVE 230 CALS**
2 slices turkey bacon	2 slices pork bacon	**25**
200g pork tenderloin	200g pork chop	**200**
A handful of pinto beans	A large handful of refried beans	**SAVE 135 CALS**

CASE STUDY

Tim Ursell's love of rugby gave him the resolve to tackle flab – follow his story if you're also looking for a conversion

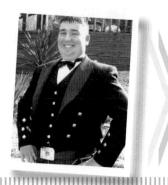

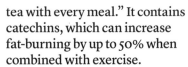

"FAT KICKED ME OFF THE TEAM"

Tim loved being playing rugby at university. But he let beer-fuelled post-match celebrations get the better of him. "I was eventually dropped from the team," says Tim. "My coach said I was 'fat and unfit'." It was the ultimate wake-up call for a man who lived for sport and it was just the motivation that Tim needed to lose weight.

"I decided to get back into the side by getting back into shape. So I started by running three times a week." Once his exercise regime was underway Tim turned his attention to his diet. "I banned sugary foods like chocolate, and drank green tea with every meal." It contains catechins, which can increase fat-burning by up to 50% when combined with exercise.

"Eating lamb's liver helped me massively," says Tim. The iron in liver helps transport more oxygenated blood to your muscles, which helps you to exercise harder.

KEEP PUSHING

As the weight dropped off Tim upped his cardio. In any weight-loss regime it's important to keep challenging yourself. If you keep exercising at beginner level, your weight loss will stall. "I'd run up to eight miles, three days a week, using hills as much as possible," says Tim. Hill running is a form of interval training – a proven fat-burner. Tim also used free weights to speed up his weight loss. No workout regime should neglect weight training. It builds muscle, which helps to burn more fat by raising your basal metabolic rate (the speed at which you burn calories when you are resting) and increases levels of testosterone.

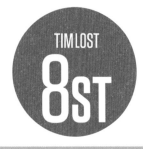

TIM LOST

8ST

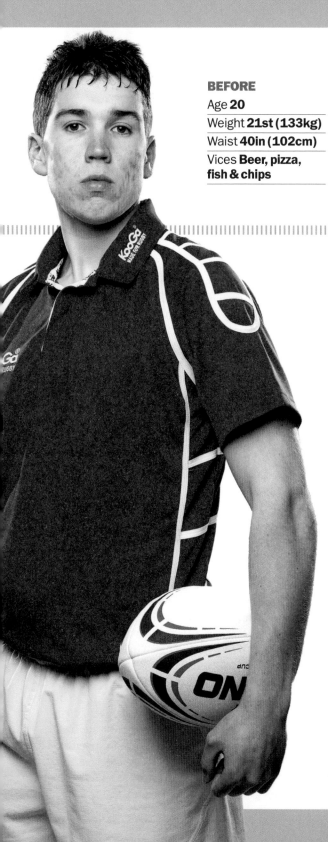

BEFORE	AFTER
Age **20**	Age **21**
Weight **21st (133kg)**	Weight **13st (82kg)**
Waist **40in (102cm)**	Waist **30in (76.2cm)**
Vices **Beer, pizza, fish & chips**	Victories **Back on the team, more confidence**

DRINK AWAY WEIGHT

The final piece of the weight loss jigsaw for Tim wasn't food or exercise… it was drink. "I hit a plateau at 16st (100kg) but giving up booze helped me to get over it," he says. One thing you should never cheat on is staying hydrated. "I got into the habit of drinking an ice-cold half-litre of water an hour before I went to bed." says Tim. Water helps suppress appetite and promotes weight loss, so make sure you keep yourself hydrated with at least two litres a day.

If you can't resist the odd tipple, it is possible to drink and lose weight – just ditch the beer and stick to wine or spirits and go for low-calorie mixers like slimline tonic or soda water.

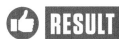 **RESULT**

"After nine months I reached my target of 13st (82kg). To keep the weight off I'm doing rugby training three times a week." Time-tabling a regular sports session is a great way to ensure you never skip workouts.

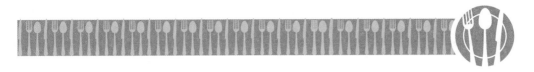

FAT-BURNING
SUPERFOODS
FOR EVERY BODY

> **LOSING WEIGHT ISN'T SIMPLY ABOUT EATING LESS, MORE IMPORTANT IS EATING *RIGHT***

YOUR REFRIGERATOR IS TO LOSING WEIGHT as a fisherman's tackle box is to catching fish. Here's how: if a fisherman is out on a lake and the trout happen to be feeding on mayflies, but he doesn't have a lure resembling a mayfly in his tackle box, he's probably not going to catch any trout. Likewise, if you're hungry but the only stuff in your fridge is a pork pie, some chocolate cake and four Stella, you're not going to advance your weight-loss efforts. A well-stocked refrigerator is like a well-appointed tackle box. It prepares you with options. And having lots of smart food options is essential in the quest to flatten your belly. There was a time when we could blame bad food choices on the people who fed us: mum, that dinner lady with the net on her head, Colonel Sanders and Ronald McDonald. Not anymore. We're adults now and free to make intelligent selections. Free to put whatever we want in that fridge.

THE PROBLEM HERE IS THAT THERE'S something attached to us that influences our food choices: a tongue. A tongue that's covered in taste buds. Therefore, we tend to eat whatever tastes good, even though it might not be good for us. The tongue, as you may have heard, is one of the most powerful muscles in the body. But there's one that's stronger: your brain. You'd be forgiven for thinking that the solution is to use willpower and get your brain to stop your tongue craving food completely: the less food you eat, the thinner you'll be. But this is actually a recipe for weight gain. Starvation diets never work. Here's why: starving yourself may cause quick weight loss at first – but fasting actually decreases the activity of enzymes that release fat from the cells. Essentially you are forcing your body to hang onto fat for all its worth. You're forcing it to think there's a famine on, so conserving resources is a natural survival response. What's more, when your body thinks there's a famine on, you're more likely to crave high-energy, sugary foods. And so you end up gaining even more weight.

Instead, the way to use your brain aid you quest for weight loss is to fill it with knowledge of good, healthy foods and listen to it. This way you don't actually have to overpower that lustful tongue, just direct it towards the foods that will aid weight loss, rather than hinder it. This chapter will help you to do just that. It contains a list of some of the healthiest foods in the world. Many of these superfoods will directly aid your body in its fight against fat and help stoke your metabolism (your fat-burning furnace). Others will help in your battle against flab indirectly by delivering optimum energy for your workouts, or boosting your immune system to reduce the chances that you'll be laid up with a cold and binge on comfort food. They will all help to ward off the ravages of ageing and more serious disease, so that, once you've hit your target weight you'll not only look great, but you'll feel great, too. Eating is an adventure in discipline and discernment. Get to know good food and how to use it. Let your adventure begin here.

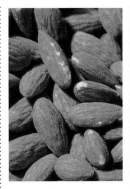

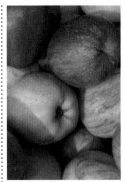

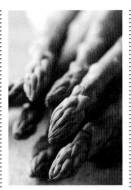

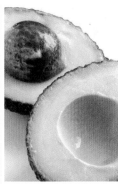

ALMONDS

Almonds on their own are an excellent weight-loss superfood, but they can get a little dry and boring. So try almond butter instead. This little-known and much under-appreciated spread, could be a star player in your larder. Try Meridian Almond Butter (£2.39, tesco.com). Check the ingredient list. It won't take long. "Almonds, 99.5%, salt 0.5%" That's it. Almond butter is a terrific spread for toast and celery sticks. A two-tablespoon serving delivers 4g of satiating fibre and 7g of protein. Of its 16g of total fat, just 1g is saturated. But watch your serving size if you are watching calories. Two tablespoons equals 195 calories. You don't need much almond butter to satisfy your hunger: which is the precisely the reason it will keep your belly at bay.

APPLES

One apple contains literally hundreds of phytochemicals, which are cholesterol-lowering and cancer-fighting nutrients. Eat the skin. Depending on the variety, apple peels have up to six times more antioxidants than the flesh alone. There's truth to the saying that one a day will keep the doctor away. Researchers in Finland found that people who regularly eat apples are 27 percent less likely to develop prediabetes and 25 percent less likely to have a stroke. Eating one apple before a meal can help you lose weight, too. Pennsylvania State University researchers found that people who ate an apple about 15 minutes before lunch consumed almost 190 fewer calories than when they didn't eat an apple. Unfortunately toffee apples don't count.

ASPARAGUS

An excellent source of folate, which helps your body to produce new blood cells. In addition, it is one of the richest sources of rutin, a compound that strengthens capillary walls. Improving blood flow and function will help you to improve your endurance so you can work out for longer and burn more fat. What's more a 150g serving delivers 3g of hunger-killing dietary fibre. If you haven't tried grilled asparagus, you're missing a real treat, and making it couldn't be easier. Just brush some olive oil over the stalks after snapping off the tough ends, and grill for about five minutes, turning often to avoid charring. Top with black pepper and sea salt. Eat them on their own as a snack or starter or as a delicious side dish.

AVOCADO

These are a great tool for weight loss because they're high in monounsaturated fats, which help to speed up your basal metabolic rate (simply put, the rate at which you can digest food). The high fat content also means you get a quick feeling of fullness, which will help prevent overeating. A study published in the *Journal of Nutrition* found that the increase in fat-burning ability prompted by monounsaturated fats was greatest for men who had a high waist-to-hip ratio, so the more belly you have to lose, the more avocados will help to burn. They are also high in beta-sitosterol, a compound that has been shown to lower cholesterol. Mix avocado with mashed, boiled egg (another fat-fighting super food) for a delicious sandwich filling.

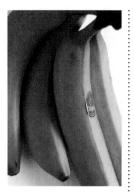

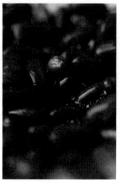

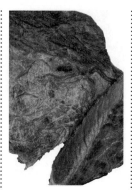

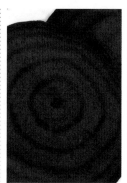

BANANAS

An excellent source of vitamin B6, which helps reduce fatigue, along with energy-giving carbohydrates, these are the perfect fruit to eat before a workout. Bananas also have a low glycaemic index, meaning even if you're not working out less of their energy will be stored as fat. Another good reason to keep a bunch to hand is that they have a creamy texture often associated with fatty foods, yet they are virtually fat free (the US Department of Agriculture reports that a large, ripe banana contains less than half a gram of fat) so they're a good way to satisfy a sweet tooth without resorting to a chocolate bar. They even fight depression and the pain of a hangover, but you're not drinking during your weight-loss regime, are you?

BEANS

One of the healthiest sources of slow-burning carbs, fibre and protein – three essentials in any fat-burning diet – beans are worthy of a spot on your daily menu. Variety makes that possible. Here's what the individual types offer.

Black beans Rich in antioxidants called anthocyanins, which fight heart disease and cancer.

Kidney beans Rich in thiamin (vitamin B1), which protects memory and brain function. Use in chilli or spaghetti sauce.

Haricot beans These are the type used in baked beans. They contain potassium, which helps to aid restful sleep: an important part of any weight-loss regime.

Pinto beans Rich in fibre, which helps stabilise blood sugar, lowering the risk of type 2 diabetes. Also a great source of energy and protein.

BEEF

A prime source of protein and rich in two other key muscle-building nutrients: iron and zinc. The more muscle you build, the faster your body will burn calories, even when it's resting, so beef is brilliant for weight loss. Plus, it's a great food source of creatine, which will helps to drive more fluid into your muscles, enabling you to lift more in the gym and build still more muscle. Yet another weight-loss bonus comes from the fact that protein takes a long time to digest, so it will make you feel fuller for longer and burn yet more calories in the process. Choose leaner cuts like sirloin or topside to reduce saturated fat intake. Cook it rare or medium to preserve nutrients and avoid burnt meat which some studies show is carcinogenic.

BEETROOT

This red vegetable is a powerhouse of folate and betaine. These two nutrients work in tandem to lower your blood levels of homocysteine, an inflammatory compound that can damage your arteries and increase your risk of heart disease. You'll reap more antioxidant benefits by eating fresh beetroot rather than their pickled cousins. Grate them into a salad. Beetroot is great for improving endurance, according to studies from the University of Exeter. They found that when volunteers drank 500ml of beetroot juice, they could cycle for an extra 92 seconds – a gift for fat burners everywhere. Beetroots in small quantities are also great for getting a decent portion of fibre – great for helping to maintain the feeling of fullness and staving off hunger.

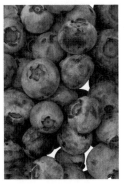

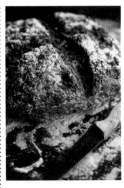

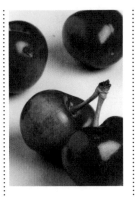

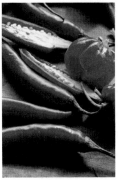

BLUEBERRIES

Try to eat a handful of these every day. Frozen ones are just as nutritious as fresh. They are packed with antioxidants and flavonoids, and contain some potassium. One particular antioxidant, pterostilbene, which is similar to the resveratrol in grapes, can stimulate liver cells to better break down fat and cholesterol, according to USDA scientists. Blueberries also fight inflammation, the key driver of many chronic diseases. Tip: The darker the berry, the more good stuff it contains, so keep an eye out for variations in colour when you're next at the supermarket. Also try strawberries, cranberries, raspberries and blackberries. They all contain decent amounts of fibre, vitamins and antioxidants.

BREAD

Whenever you eat bread, make sure it's wholemeal. White bread has no place in the lean man's larder – it will spike your blood sugar levels and have you craving more carbs within the hour. On the other hand bread made with wholemeal flour will provide slow-release energy that will keep you feeling fuller for longer. Other ways to lower the GI of your loaf even further are to look out for seeded varieties, or even ones containing sprouted-grain. They may contain more calories per slice, but the satiating effects of those added extras will be worth it. A couple of slices of decent wholemeal bread is lower in calories than a comparable wholemeal wrap, so use your loaf and roll out the sandwiches.

CHERRIES

Regular sweet cherries have more antioxidants per serving than red grapes, edamame, or carrots. Antioxidants are known to help prevent stroke and slow the signs of ageing. However, more importantly from a fat-burning perspective, they will also help to bolster your immune system, meaning you are less likely to come down with a nasty cold which could knock out your gym routine and have you craving sugary comfort food. The anti-inflammatory compounds in cherries may help lower the risk of heart disease as well as arthritis and cancer. If you can't be doing with stones, cherries also make very good juice – but stay away from the added-sugar 'juice drink' varieties, which will derail weight loss.

CHILLIES

Poblanos, serranos, habaneros, jalapeños... all chillies contain a compound called capsaicin, which gives them their spicy heat and serves to fire up your metabolism, ensuring that your body is always on top fat-burning form. This happens through a process called thermogenesis – heat creation – which means our bodies burn up calories to warm us up rather than storing them. This is why you sweat when you have a hot curry. Chillis are also high in carotene and flavonoids and contain more than twice the amount of vitamin C found in citrus fruits, all of which will help to bolster you immune system. Using chillies in low-fat foods can help satisfy our cravings for oily food and stop us from feeling hungry later.

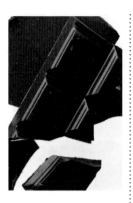 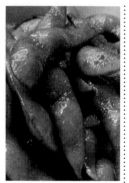 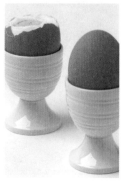 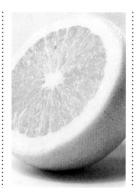

CHOCOLATE

No, not the milky variety, filled with caramel. We're talking dark chocolate here, with a high percentage of cocoa solids. Milk blocks the absorption of chocolate's antioxidants, so the lighter variety isn't worth the calories you'll have to take on. The darker the chocolate, the more antioxidant flavonols and the less sugar it has. Watch out, though: some manufacturers up the percentage of cocoa by adding extra cocoa butter. When selecting yours, always keep an eye on saturated fat counts. A study in the US *Archives of Internal Medicine* found that eating a small amount of dark chocolate regularly aids weight loss. This is thought to be due to the fact that it reduces cravings for other sweet foods, so you'll be less likely to go on a binge.

EDAMAME

These little wonders are often served as a starter or side dish in Asian cuisine. They're actually baby soybeans still in their pods and as such are a terrific way to boost fibre and protein while keeping saturated fat levels extremely low. A study conducted at the University of Illinois found that increasing soy protein intake aids fat burning. What's more a separate study published in the *Journal of the American Medical Association* showed that a diet containing soy protein lowered cholesterol as much as statins, the most widely prescribed cholesterol medicine. These make a great start to any meal as they will increase feelings of satiety. They also make a great alternative to snacking on crisps. Keep some in a bowl on your desk.

EGGS

There's a reason Rocky drank six uncooked eggs before training: they are high in muscle-building protein and important B vitamins. While you don't have to down so many of them raw, it's worth considering them as your default breakfast. A study of 30 overweight people found that those who ate two scrambled eggs with two slices of wholemeal toast in the morning consumed less for the next 36 hours than those who had a bagel breakfast of equal calories. Part of the reason for this is thought to be that their protein helps prevent spikes in blood sugar, which can lead to food cravings. Never have more than two egg yolks a day, however, as the high cholesterol levels in them can be harmful to your health.

GRAPEFRUIT

A study by the Nutrition and Metabolic Research Centre at Scripps clinic in the US showed that people who added half a grapefruit to each of their normal meals lost a minimum of 3.6lb (1.6kg) over a 12-week period, though many lost much more. Grapefruit reduces insulin spikes and thus encourages weight loss. Sprinkle with brown sugar, add a dash of angostura bitters and put under a grill for a few minutes. The red or pink varieties are slightly higher in vitamin C than the white. They also contain lycopene, which may reduce the risk of prostate cancer. But all varieties have natural compounds called limonoids, which can lower cholesterol. If you're not having eggs for breakfast you should probably have grapefruit instead.

GREEN TEA

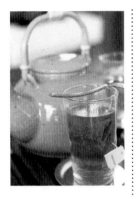

A recent study at Fudan University in China showed that catechins – antioxidants found in green tea – can help the body to burn fat. Having a daily brew for 12 weeks was enough to see a significant boost to weight-loss efforts. Not only that but green tea is packed with other disease-fighting antioxidants and, contrary to popular belief, is actually quite high in caffeine, so is a good way to boost your energy levels before a workout. Green tea comes in a variety of flavours, including citrus, cranberry and jasmine – so even if you don't like the regular stuff, you can probably find an alternative that will suit your tastes. Try making a large pot and putting it in the fridge to cool for a fat-zapping alternative to sugary fizzy drinks.

GREEN VEG

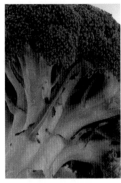

Leafy greens from the cabbage family, also known as cruciferous vegetables (such as broccoli, brussels sprouts, cauliflower, cabbage, kale and bok choi) contain cancer-fighting phytochemicals, vitamin C, fibre, and folate. Although they are technically carbohydrate, levels are low as is their GI, so you can pile you plate high and never have to worry about weight gain. The filling effects of the fibre should also stop you craving more calorific alternatives. Consumption of these vegetables seem to be associated with reduced rates of cancers of the lung, colon, prostate and bladder because of chemicals that activate detoxification enzymes in the body. Eat them steamed or raw to retain the nutrients.

HUMMUS

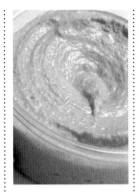

This spread made of mashed chickpeas, tahini and olive oil is rich in protein and fibre. The tahini, a paste made of ground sesame seeds, delivers omega-3 fatty acids. You don't need to eat much; it's filling and high in calories, but it makes a great high-fibre, high-protein alternative to mayonnaise in sandwiches. You can also get a variety of different flavours such as garlic hummus and red pepper hummus, so you should never get bored. When you're not eating hummus you can still toss chickpeas into a salad. They can help slash LDL ("bad") cholesterol levels by almost 5 percent. Try adding spicy chilli powder or paprika to your hummus to give your metabolism an extra boost. See 'Chillies' to find out why.

KIWIS

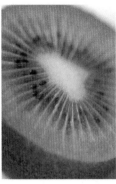

A good source of vitamin C and fibre, Kiwis also contain as much potassium as bananas, and are full of antioxidants. Despite being furry, the skins are full of nutrients, so throwing them in to a smoothie is a great way to get the most out of them. Kiwis are also a little-known source of omega-3 fatty acids. A recent study at the University of South Australia found consuming omega-3s and undertaking an exercise regime led to an average 4.5lb (2kg) of extra weight loss compared to subjects who exercised but did not consume omega-3s. Kiwi has also been linked to cleaning the body of toxins and removing harmful chemicals and substances from the bloodstream. Eat them halved with a spoon, or whole… if you dare.

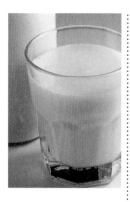
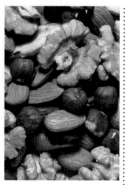
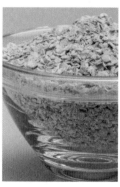
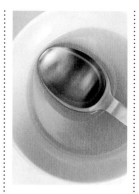

MILK

The beautiful thing about milk is that it has substance, so it helps you feel satisfied quickly and forestalls bingeing. Just skip the Maryland cookies, or you'll have a nutritional mutiny on your hands. Here's another terrific thing about milk. A University of Tennessee study found that dieters who consumed between 1,200 and 1,300mg of calcium a day lost nearly twice as much weight as those taking in less calcium. Another study in the *Journal of the American College of Nutrition*, which surveyed 1,300 people ages 19-38, concluded that increasing intake of calcium and low-fat dairy products may be associated with lower amounts of abdominal fat, particularly in young men. Milk is also good for strengthening bones so you'll be less injury prone.

NUTS

In a study of more than 3,000 African-American men and women, those who ate nuts at least five times a week cut their risk of dying of heart disease by 44 percent compared with people who ate nuts less frequently. Most nuts are the perfect snack food, packed with muscle-building protein, filling fibre, and heart-healthy fats. Numerous studies have shown that almonds, Brazil nuts, hazelnuts, macadamia nuts, pecans, pistachios and walnuts all reduce levels of LDL cholesterol. Devouring bags of dry roasted at the local boozer won't do your waist any favours, though. Substitute them for some raw pistachios to get the fibre and protein you need to keep you feeling full without the unhealthy, salty coating.

OATS

It's hard to find a better breakfast. Porridge will fill you up with long-burning clean energy. In fact, Pennsylvania State University researchers found that oats keep insulin levels stable longer than most other foods, which means you won't find yourself craving chocolate bars an hour after you eat. You have a couple of choices when it comes to oats. Steel-cut oats contain more fibre because they are thicker cut, resulting in a chewier oatmeal that's less processed than rolled oats. They'll keep you fuller longer, but they take longer to prepare. If you are pressed for time, the instant oatmeal (rolled oats) is a lot more convenient. Choose the unsweetened, unflavoured variety to avoid a lot of unnecessary sugar.

OLIVE OIL

This staple of the famously healthy Mediterranean diet is a powerhouse food that controls cravings, helps burn fat, and can even build muscle. Olive oil contains monounsaturated fat that has been associated with everything from lower rates of heart disease and colon cancer to a reduced risk of diabetes and osteoporosis. You've heard about that for years, but what you may not know is that it also appears to prevent muscle breakdown by lowering levels of a cellular protein that is linked to muscle wasting and weakness. Choose extra-virgin olive oil, which has higher levels of vitamin E. Cook with it or dress salads to satisfy cravings for fatty foods in a healthy way. Don't overdo it though, fat is still high in calories.

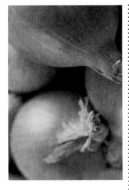

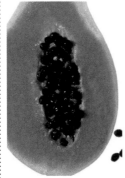

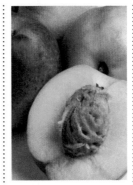

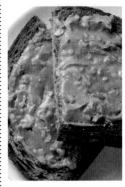

ONIONS

You can add garlic, chives, spring onions and shallots to this entry as these breath busters are all cousins, belonging to the alliaceous family. The sulfur compounds found in them fight colon and lung cancers and studies show that people who consume the most garlic and onions have a lower risk of stomach, colorectal and prostate cancers. The active compounds in garlic are released when you crush the clove, and they become more robust when sautéed in a little olive oil. Onions contain chromium, an organic compound that helps your body to respond to insulin, and assists in regulating blood sugar so reducing food cravings between meals. Onions are also quite high in fibre, so will help to fill you up without skimping on flavour.

PAPAYAS

If you have a cold, eat a papaya. One medium papaya delivers more than 300 percent of your RDA of vitamin C. Each papaya also contains two-thirds of your RDA of vitamin A, useful for boosting immunity and eye health. When it comes to weight loss the papaya has a secret weapon as it contains papain, a unique enzyme that helps digest proteins. This compound is helpful for weight loss as it makes muscle-building protein more accessible to your body. The more muscle you have the more calories you will need to burn, even when you are sitting around doing nothing. What's more papayas will even help you recover from your workout as their beta-carotene and vitamins C and E help to reduce inflammation throughout the body.

PEACHES

A solid source of vitamin C for healthy skin and immune system, peaches also have a good amount of dietary fibre to help promote digestive health and keep you feeling full. Peaches also have a higher vitamin C content than oranges, and are low on the glycaemic index, meaning they are turned into glucose – your body's energy source – slowly. Skip the canned varieties, as the syrup they come in is full of calorific sugar, and stops them from being healthy. Instead try slicing a fresh one on top of your cereal in the morning, or simply take one to work as a snack. The sugars in them are natural and healthy, nevertheless you should avoid peaches late at night as you won't have time to burn off their energy.

PEANUTS

Getting your peanuts in butter form is an easy way to consume this superfood daily. Go for no-added sugar versions such as Whole Earth (£2.69, tesco.com), that way you'll avoid unnecessary calories. Peanut butter is full of heart-healthy fats and protein, both of which will keep you feeling fuller for longer. It also contains a high amount of monounsaturated fats, similar to those contained in olive oil, so can help to reduce cholesterol and lower your risk of heart attack. A study from Purdue University in the US found that when people of normal-weight added about 500 calories worth of peanuts to their diet, they consumed less at subsequent meals. It also revved up their resting metabolism by as much as 11%.

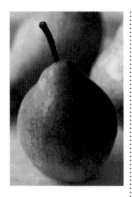

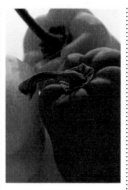

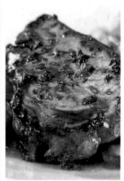

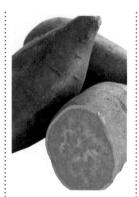

PEARS

This tasty and nutrient-rich fruit is a top source of fibre, vitamin C, and folate, which together can help lower cholesterol, build immunity to infection – vital if you want to ensure you don't get sidelined from the gym by a nasty cold. To get the most from them, eat the skin as well, as this is where most of the filling fibre and other nutrients are. Pears are delicious chopped into some yoghurt or mixed in with porridge. Because pears are full of fibre, they can help you stay full and satiated throughout the day and prevent craving for sweets and biscuits. Eating a pear as a snack in mid-morning or mid-afternoon between meals can be a good way to get vitamins and minerals as well as stay full and prevent cravings for more unhealthy snacks.

PEPPERS

Red, green, yellow, and orange – all are good sources of vitamins, including the hard-to-get vitamin B6, which will help to ensure optimum energy levels. They contain lots of organic phytochemicals that can protect you from heart disease, cancer, stroke and even cataracts. At as little as 24 calories for a medium green pepper, these tasty little beauties can be added to salads, chilli, wraps or sauces to give them their peppery taste. Like their spicier cousins, peppers are good for kick-starting your metabolism because they contain capsaicin, although not as much as the jalapeño or super-hot scotch bonnet. Peppers contain a lot of water and fibre – also useful components in weight loss. Slice them into a salad or stuff them with brown rice.

PORK CHOPS

Researchers have found that a serving of pork daily helped people that worked out preserve their muscle while losing weight. Pork chops contain a large amount of protein relative to their size, which makes them good for keeping your metabolism going and for building muscle. Normal supermarket-bought pork chops do contain quite a bit of fat, though, so it's really important to cut the fat from them if you can, and to avoid pigging out. These are great grilled with a little extra virgin olive oil and a healthy rocket salad. Or slice them into strips and use in a healthy stir fry. Per gram of protein, pork chops contain almost five times the selenium – an essential mineral that's linked to a lower risk of prostate cancer – of beef, and twice that of chicken.

POTATOES

While regular potatoes are a lot better for you than refined carbs such as bread and pasta, if you really want a superfood you need to go for sweet potatoes. They are higher in fibre than white potatoes and also have a low GI, so they'll provide slow-release energy and keep you feeling fuller for longer. What's more European researchers recently found pigments from beta-carotene-rich foods such as sweet potatoes and carrots can build up in your skin, helping to prevent ultraviolet rays from ageing skin. They are great roasted, boiled or even microwaved. Mashed with a little olive oil, sweet potatoes can be a good side dish with some grilled chicken or steak. Sweet potato wedges are also a tasty alternative to chips, but go easy on the salt.

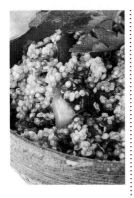

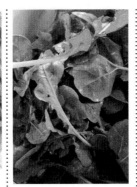

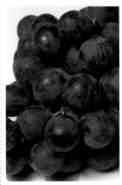

QUINOA

Quinoa (pronounced Keen-wa) is usually called a grain, but is actually closely related to leafy veg such as spinach and swiss chard. Quinoa has about twice the protein of regular cereal grains, as well as fewer carbohydrates and even some healthy fats. It's considered a "complete" protein, like eggs, because it contains all the essential amino acids your body needs for muscle growth: don't forget how important muscle growth is for weight loss. Quinoa can be used to make pilafs, risottos, salads, and soups. Because of its high levels of protein and fibre, it can help you feel full and satisfied. Originally from South America, this supergrain has been called 'the mother of all grains'. Find it in the rice aisle of your local supermarket.

RICE

Here's why you should choose brown rice over white rice at every opportunity: the milling and polishing process that converts brown rice into white rice destroys 80 percent of the thiamin, 80 percent of the niacin, half of the B6, 75 percent of the magnesium, 60 percent of the iron, and nearly all of the dietary fibre. For brown rice, only the outermost layer of the hull of the kernel is removed, so it suffers the least damage to its nutritional value. You know that whole grains like brown rice are satiating, but the high fibre content of brown rice also favorably affects blood glucose levels, which is important for weight loss. The latest research shows that men who eat brown rice generally weigh up to 1.1kg less than men who eat white rice.

ROCKET

Nothing against the venerable head of iceberg lettuce, but there are other foundations on which to build a nutritious salad. Peppery-flavoured rocket is one of them; it contains about twice as much bone-building calcium and magnesium as iceberg. Other ways to extend your leafy green repertoire: romaine, red leaf and green leaf lettuces; spinach; watercress; red chard and radicchio. For an easy path into unfamiliar salad-green territory, buy a package of spring mix, which contains many of the above. Rocket is nearly entirely calorie-free, meaning you could burn more calories preparing it than you get from eating it. Perfect. You can throw it into sandwiches, salads, pasta and pizzas. It's not difficult, but it is, in fact, rocket science.

RED GRAPES

Besides providing protection from heart attack and stroke, antioxidants in red grapes may also help keep your skin flexible and elastic. The resveratrol in red grape skins may help prevent colon cancer, according to researchers at the University of California. Grapes are low in calories, easy to eat without preparation and very tasty. Most of the calories in grapes are in the form of fructose, a sugar easily turned into energy by our body. Grapes help to reduce levels of LDLs ('bad' cholesterol) in our bodies, helping to reduce the risk of heart attack and stroke. Raisins (which are simply dried grapes) contain the same levels of resveratrol, and are great in your porridge. Try freezing a few grapes for a refreshing snack on a hot day.

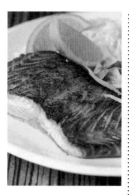
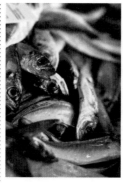
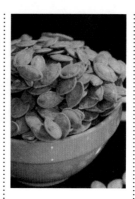
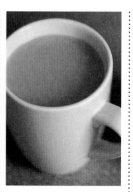

SALMON

This fish is rich in the omega-3 fatty acid DHA. People with the highest blood levels of this nutrient have a 47 percent lower chance of developing dementia, according to a study published in the Archives of Neurology. DHA, a component of neurons, plays a key role in memory and learning. It's best to eat wild salmon rather than farmed fish; the farmed salmon may not get the appropriate marine diet needed to produce high amounts of omega-3s. The low level of dangerous saturated fat in salmon means it's a great replacement for your usual portion of red meat such as steak. Salmon is a tasty way to get a filing fix on protein while keeping calories under control, so try it with spinach and steamed broccoli, or see the recipe in Chapter Seven.

SARDINES

This delicious cold-water fish delivers some of the highest amounts of omega-3 fatty acids and protein of any food. Not only is fish oil an anti-inflammatory agent, it also helps protect against heart arrhythmias. And a single can of sardines has more calcium than a cup of whole milk (because you eat the bones). Omega-3s help suppress the activity of prostaglandins and leukotrienes, which can activate various diseases, including blood clots and joint inflammation. Omega-3s also help protect the immune system. Sardines in oil are often higher in fat and calories than those in brine, so choose carefully. Try grilling or cooking into a pasta sauce instead of some higher-calorie meats to get your fix of omega-3.

SEEDS

Pumpkin seeds Roasted, pumpkin seeds contain 150mg of magnesium per 30g serving. That's over a third of your RDA, so sprinkle them on your cereal every morning. Eat them whole; the shells provide extra fibre, which will keep you feeling full and ward off snack attacks.

Flaxseeds Flaxseeds contain the highest percentage of omega-3 of any plant product. Toss them into cereal, yoghurt, soups, and stews, and sprinkle them on top of ice cream. Researchers have suggested that they may even aid in the reduction of cholesterol.

Sunflower seeds If you want to look younger, eat sunflower seeds. They have the highest natural vitamin E content of any food around, which will help to improve the condition of your skin and functioning of your eyes.

TEA

Your classic cup of builders is packed with disease-fighting antioxidants and it is also an extremely low-calorie beverage with a small hit of caffeine, which will help to keep your metabolism ticking over – a perfect recipe for weight loss. Switch from milk and two sugars to an artificial zero-calorie sweetener and skimmed milk to cut down the bad bits. Or, why not take a leaf out of our American cousin's pot and drink it iced on hot days? All you have to do is make a pot, pour it out into a bottle before it gets too stewed, then let it cool and then stick it in the fridge. It will keep well for a few days and makes a great replacement for sugary fizzy drinks, poured over ice. Tea itself is calorie-free, so it's like water with extra benefits. Go on. Stick the kettle on.

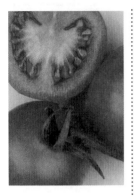

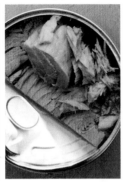

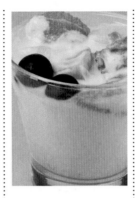

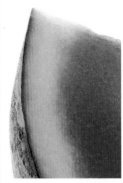

TOMATOES

According to America's Food and Drug Administration, eating tomatoes may reduce the risk of prostate, gastric and pancreatic cancers, thanks to their high concentration of the antioxidant lycopene. What's more, preparing food with fresh tomatoes usually means you are going to get a lot of other fresh, healthy ingredients in there, so they should be a staple in your fridge. Tomatoes also contain key organic compounds that can help to stimulate your metabolism. Tomato juice is almost as good as the actual things, so try starting your day with a Virgin Mary. You'll not only get the nutritious benefit of the tomatoes, the Tabasco will help to give your metabolism an extra boost thanks to the capsaicinoids, which make it taste hot.

TUNA

This low-fat fish is a great protein source, which is essential for muscle building. What makes it an even better weight loss food, however, is the fact that it is full of vitamins B6 and B12, which aid digestion as well as reducing stress. Research from the University of Maryland School of Medicine in the US found that the cortisol released when you're under pressure sends messages to your body to refuel itself, even if it doesn't need to. Basically stress makes you hungry. The B vitamins found in tuna will help to counteract this effect. So next time you're under the kosh, hit the gym at lunch for some feel-good endorphins, then refuel with a tuna salad. You'll avoid dashing out for a chocolate bar in the afternoon.

YOGHURT

Yoghurt is one of the few foods that contain conjugated linoleic acid, a special type of fat that some studies show can reduces body fat. And if you're exercising hard, this stuff delivers a perfect combination of protein and carbohydrates for workout recovery and muscle growth. High in calcium and important B-vitamins, yoghurt should be the basis of many low-fat weight loss recipes. Adding in dried fruit, nuts or granola can add texture to your yoghurt. Replacing a mid-afternoon snack or your breakfast with a portion of yoghurt can help to drop a few extra pounds. You can even freeze a large tub to get a tasty alternative to ice-cream, with half the fat. Check the packs before buying, some low-fat yoghurts add extra sugar.

WATERMELON

One large wedge provides 250ml of water. Keeping yourself hydrated is extremely important in your battle against fat. People who are thirsty often misinterpret the sensation for hunger and end up overeating instead of drinking. A slice of watermelon will also help to satisfy a sweet tooth, for minimal calorie damage – making it an almost perfect weight loss food. High in citrulline, watermelon is great as a post-workout snack or sports drink replacement during a workout. Citrulline is shown to help reduce muscle fatigue, meaning you can exercise for longer, burning more fat. You can freeze watermelon and eat it like a sorbet for an extremely low-calorie and healthy dessert, or have a wedge for breakfast – there's no bad time for watermelon.

HOW TO UP FIBRE INTAKE TO
FIGHT FAT
15 WAYS TO GET MORE OF THIS FILLING NUTRIENT

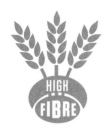

You Guideline Daily Amount of fibre is 24g. It's an excellent nutrient to have more of when you are trying to lose weight as it fills you up for very few calories. However, it can be pretty tough to get that much fibre in a typical diet. But you can come really close to, if not hit, those numbers without thinking much and certainly without counting. Just make a handful of these tricks everyday habits.

1 Drop in a handful of berries to add flavour to plain or vanilla yoghurt. A handful will provide around 4g of fibre.

2 Pile on the vegetables by layering your sandwich with fresh spinach, tomatoes, sprouts, cucumbers, or peppers.

3 Add roughage to dips by mixing some blended kidney beans

4 Choose 100 percent wholemeal bread for a sandwich, and you'll add 3-5g of fibre per serving.

5 Toss ground flaxseeds onto salads or soups for extra bulk and heart-friendly omega-3s.

6 Blend a handful of fresh or frozen fruit into a smoothie. Leave the skins on for up to 4g of fibre.

7 Snack on a small bowl of popcorn for 2g of fibre.

8 Sprinkle garbanzo beans on your salad. A small handfu delivers up to 6g of extra fibre.

9 Use raw carrots, broccoli, or pepper strips for dipping, rather than crisps.

10 Stir a fibre supplement containing psyllium into water or juice twice a day, and you'll get an easy 5g.

11 Crunch on about 30g of almonds, peanuts, cashews or pecans for 2-4g of fibre.

12 Top salads or cooked vegetables with crushed bran cereal or unprocessed wheat bran for an additional 3.5g of fibre.

13 For dessert, eat dried figs, apricots, or peaches. Add nuts for a fibre-packed trail mix.

14 Bite an apple, then spread on some almond butter or crunchy natural peanut butter where you just bit. Bite, spread. Repeat.

15 Eat the skin of your next baked potato for an extra 2g of fibre.

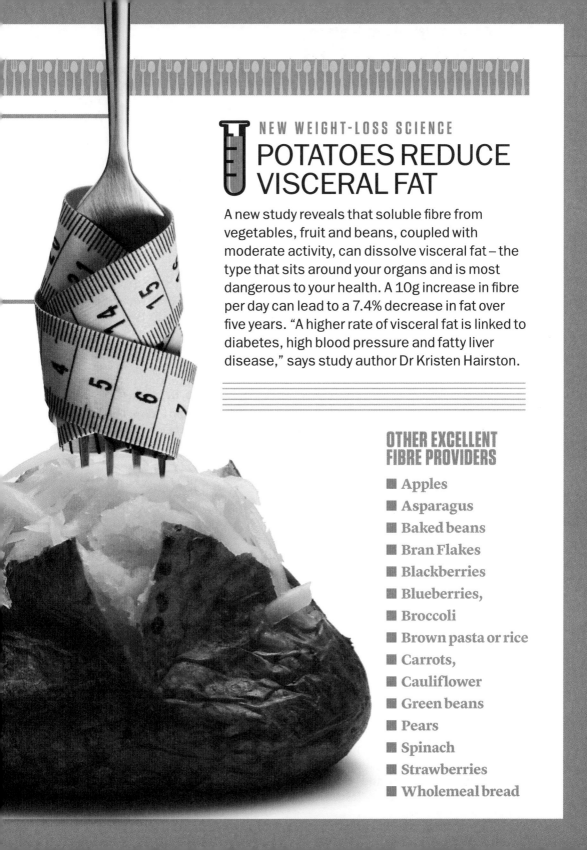

NEW WEIGHT-LOSS SCIENCE

POTATOES REDUCE VISCERAL FAT

A new study reveals that soluble fibre from vegetables, fruit and beans, coupled with moderate activity, can dissolve visceral fat – the type that sits around your organs and is most dangerous to your health. A 10g increase in fibre per day can lead to a 7.4% decrease in fat over five years. "A higher rate of visceral fat is linked to diabetes, high blood pressure and fatty liver disease," says study author Dr Kristen Hairston.

OTHER EXCELLENT FIBRE PROVIDERS

- Apples
- Asparagus
- Baked beans
- Bran Flakes
- Blackberries
- Blueberries,
- Broccoli
- Brown pasta or rice
- Carrots,
- Cauliflower
- Green beans
- Pears
- Spinach
- Strawberries
- Wholemeal bread

CASE STUDY

Dan Evans from Folkestone used feedback from fellow fat burners on menshealth.co.uk to almost half his body weight in just 12 months

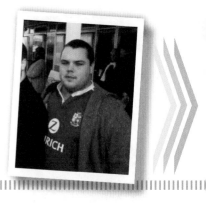

"JUST TYING MY LACES WAS HARD"

Dan Evans gained weight after a loss. "After my dad died, I put on 5st in 18 months by binge eating," says Dan. "My body fat rose to 38%. I got out of breath just tying my shoelaces and realised I was wrecking my life," says Dan. Body fat levels over 25% are officially obese, while 8-20% should be your healthy target range. Dan realised it was time to turn his life around.

"I started off with some drastic changes to my diet; ditching junk food and opting for high-protein, moderate-carb and moderate-fat intake," he says. "Meanwhile, on the exercise front I used a weekly 'rule of four' for cardio."

"Four cardiovascular workout sessions a week is optimum for stripping body fat," says strength and conditioning coach Michael Mejia. "Alternate your methods of cardio for even better results."

Next Dan hired a trainer to help with his weight loss. "He suggested compound lifts three times a week. On the days without weights I did High Intensity Interval Training (HIIT) on the rower" These are exercise drills featuring repeated bursts of intense training and are excellent for burning fat.

WEB PAGE HITS

"I logged my fat-burning progress on menshealth.co.uk/fatburnerforum and the feedback helped me tweak my routine and stay on course," says Dan. US studies show incentives such as regular emails significantly motivate people to maintain weight loss, "Top tips included eating tuna

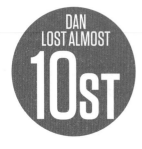

DAN LOST ALMOST **10ST**

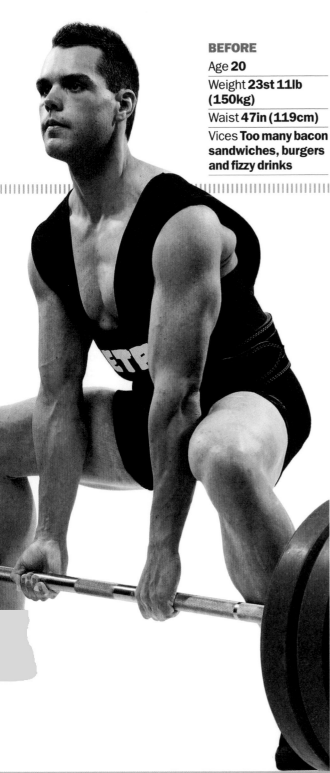

BEFORE

Age **20**

Weight **23st 11lb (150kg)**

Waist **47in (119cm)**

Vices **Too many bacon sandwiches, burgers and fizzy drinks**

AFTER

Age **21**

Weight **13.5st (84kg)**

Waist **32in (81cm)**

Victories **New love of powerlifting, first girlfriend in five years**

in chilli-infused olive oil and drinking five litres of water a day," says Dan. If the taste of fish turns you off, try a cod liver oil supplement (Seven Seas, £9.06, superliving.co.uk). Australian studies reveal they lower your body fat percentage, showing your gut no mercy. "After five months I was down to 16st (101kg)."

CYCLE OF SUCCESS

"I switched my diet to a macro carb cycle," says Dan. This is an eating plan which involves high-carb days when weight training to ensure glycogen is restored, followed by lower carb recovery days when the bulk of calories come from protein.

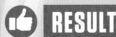 **RESULT**

"I took up powerlifting and I'm now leaner, with just 12% body fat," says Dan. Weight training stokes your metabolism by building muscle, which will burn more fat even when you are resting.

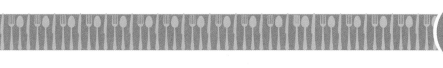

9

THE
50 BEST
FOOD TIPS

TRICKS TO HELP YOU TO BUST THROUGH
ANY WEIGHT-LOSS PLATEAUX

SMALL STEPS HOLD THE SECRET TO MAKING ANYTHING worthwhile happen, from learning to play the guitar to bouncing back from a job loss. It certainly applies to the challenges of losing weight and getting back in shape. It's not a revolutionary notion by any means. But it's clever. And it works. Have you hit a plateau? Are the pounds slower to come off these days? Are your muscles sore? Do you feel like ditching your workout and diving into stuffed-crust pizza with pepperoni? All that's normal. And that's why this chapter has 50 smart ways to turbocharge your weight-loss efforts. When it comes to cooking and eating, tiny tweaks can add up to more pounds lost and another notch on your belt.

1 Swap your regular cheese for goat's cheese. It's 40% lower in calories than cheddar.

2 Eat chilli con carne once a week. An enzyme in kidney beans tells the body to break down stored fat instead of carbs for energy, while the chillies boost your metabolism.

3 Make yourself a salad of black beans, peppers, tomatoes, onion and sweet corn with an olive oil and lemon dressing. It will help weight loss. The combination of fibre, hunger suppressants and fat-burning chemicals will to shed the pounds.

4 Chew sugar-free gum. It releases a chemical that makes us feel full, according to the *Journal of Medicinal Chemistry*.

5 Eating a bowl of muesli two hours before training increases fat burning during your session, says a study in the *International Journal of Sport Nutrition and Exercise Metabolism*.

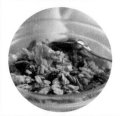

6 A daily glass of red wine can stop you putting on fat, especially around your belly. Resveratrol from the grapes inhibits the development of fat cells around your waist according to the University of Athens in Georgia.

7 When buying pork the best cut to go for is tenderloin because it has the same fat as skinless chicken, say the US Department of Agriculture.

8 Eat more berries. They contain less fructose than other fruits, which can combine with carbs to form body fat.

9 If you have cheese after a meal, choose camembert to boost fat fighting. It contains fat-burning calcium and sleep-inducing tryptophan.

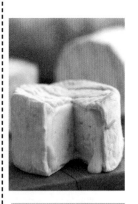

10 Choose spinach ahead of other greens. It packs double the fibre, which helps your body process fats more efficiently.

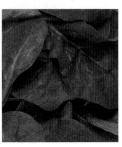

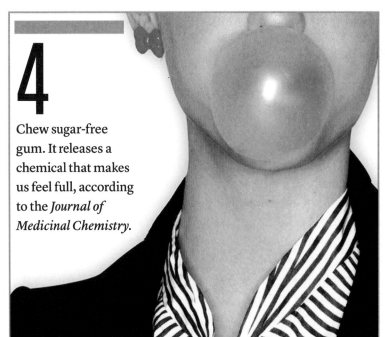

12 Putting tomatoes in your sandwiches will help you to stay feeling fuller longer. A study carried out by Imperial College London found this is because tomatoes suppress the hormone ghrelin, which is a major cause of food cravings.

13 Swap rice for grated cauliflower to shave your gut. It's non-starchy, and the vitamin C hit helps you burn body fat for fuel during physical activity.

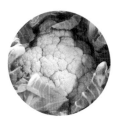

14 Sprinkle cinnamon into a yoghurt each day to burn fat. A study published in the journal *Phytomedicine* found that this spice is a powerful metabolism raiser; half a teaspoon a day is enough to burn an extra kilo a month.

11 Avoid energy drinks during your workout. Their high-GI carbs can make you pick up body fat. The high levels of caffeine also inhibit blood flow according to the *American College of Cardiology*.

15 Stress at work is the biggest cause of overeating according to the *American Journal of Clinical Nutrition*. Controlled breathing for two minutes, will dampen hunger pangs.

16 A strategic tipple aids weight loss. Small amounts of alcohol increase the body's metabolic rate, causing more calories to be burned, according to a study in the *Archives of Internal Medicine*.

17 Fire up the barbecue to grill away the calories in your meat: it's much healthier than frying or roasting because barbecuing meat lets extra fat escape during cooking.

18 No carbs at all will lead to storing more fat in the long run. So cut your carb intake by 200g a week to stimulate the appetite repressing hormone leptin and kick-start your metabolism. Swap common carbs for fibre to stay full for longer.

19 Turn off your TV while you eat. This will cut 3.5kg of weight gain each year, according to the University of Birmingham.

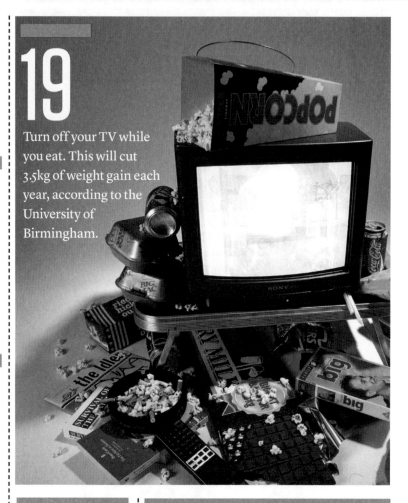

20 Eating plain popcorn lowers your blood glucose levels, helping to burn fat, according to dieticians at St George's hospital, London.

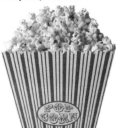

21 Eat less with acupuncture. A study in the *International Journal of Obesity* found that you could lose an extra 4.5kg in three months by having weekly acupuncture. The triggered impulses can suppress appetite.

22 Glasses with blue lenses block hunger-stimulating red light, according to the University of Nevada.

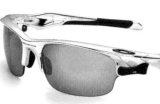

23

Hit the Horlicks before bed – it's full of sleep-inducing trytophan. Lack of sleep causes spikes in cortisol, disturbs blood sugar, and leads to overeating, according to a Mayo Clinic study.

24

Sprinkle a little olive oil on a few leaves of kale. Then bake them until crispy (about 15-20 minutes) and add spice or salt to taste. Crisps don't come healthier than this.

25

Always eat slowly. "We don't have instant feedback from our bodies," says Janet Polivy, professor of psychology at the University of Toronto. "It takes 20 minutes for food to be digested enough that glucose gets into the bloodstream and the satiety hormones start working."

26

Take a hot bath in the evenings to aid your digestion. It will also set you up for sleep, which keeps your blood sugar balanced.

27

Always eat apples and pears with their skin on, you'll get more vitamins and more fibre, which will help you to feel fuller for longer.

28

Slice your food to consume 20% fewer calories. People rate sliced servings as 27% larger than equal amounts of whole food.

29

Don't get tempted by bread baskets in restaurants. It may not cost anything, but it's not free from calories.

30

Sip green tea. It contains a compound that reacts with caffeine to boost fat oxidation and resting metabolism by 20%.

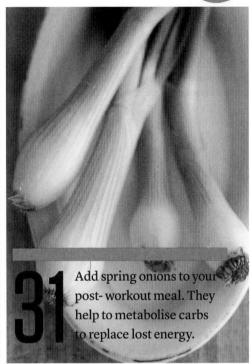

31

Add spring onions to your post-workout meal. They help to metabolise carbs to replace lost energy.

32

Order a large meal rather than a mixed platter. Small dishes encourage overeating.

33

Buy a gravy separator. It splits fat from gravy, making it healthier (£7.50, debenhams.com.)

34

Divide your food into single servings before eating to avoid overindulging.

35 Tempted by an all-you-can-eat Chinese? Cut calorie intake by 30% by using chopsticks to slow yourself down.

36 Eat more beans. A study, in the *American Journal of Clinical Nutrition* found eating any type every day makes you 23% less likely to add size to your waist.

37 Freeze bananas to use in smoothies. That way you'll always have them on hand and there'll be no need for ice.

38 A glass of carrot juice a day will help you lose 4lbs over 12 weeks, compared to non-juice drinkers. It's high in fibre and nutrients that help burn blubber.

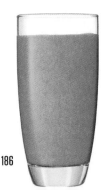

39 Lentils are one of the best weight-loss foods. They are high in filling fibre and protein. They also contain the amino acid leucine, which burns fat fast.

40 If you're making a Thai curry, replace the coconut milk with low-fat plain yoghurt. It's creamy without adding calories.

41 Eat as many different colours fruit and veg as possible for varied nutrients and faster fat-burning.

42 For perfect steaming when you're in a rush, rinse vegetables in water then throw in sealed container and microwave for 3-4 minutes.

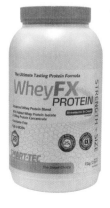

43 Take a whey protein. The University of Adelaide in Australia found that whey increases insulin sensitivity, drastically reducing you chances of contracting diabetes.

44 Sprinkle paprika on your meals. The ground red peppers in it contain around six times the vitamin C of tomatoes, crucial for helping your body to turn fat into energy.

46 One tablespoon of fresh oregano has more antioxidants than an entire apple. Antioxidants help prevent damage caused by toxins present in fats broken down during weight loss. Oregano tastes great in pasta, salads and on meats so sprinkle it on your cooking for an easy boost to your daily nutrition.

47 Eat a portion of dairy every day. The calcium in it helps to increase the rate your body metabolises fat, according to a study at the University of Tennessee.

45 Here's a great breakfast smoothie: blend 200g strawberries, 125ml soya milk and 2tsps vanilla extract. Soy contains less fat than skimmed milk, and strawberries stimulate your metabolism.

48 Drizzle on some soy sauce to shed the pounds. Research shows soy proteins interact with receptors in our brains that tell us we're full.

49 Wait before going for seconds. It takes your brain 20 minutes to tell you that you feel full.

50 A study in *The American Journal of Agricultural and Food Chemistry* found that black pepper contains piperine, which can help block the formation of new fat cells.

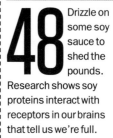

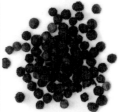

CASE STUDY

Simon Lim, from Glasgow, punched away his paunch in just 20 weeks. Here are his tips for super-fast weight loss

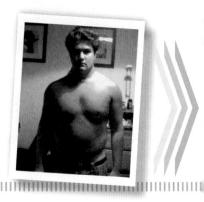

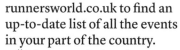

"UNIVERSITY LIFE HIT ME IN THE GUT"

The end of his student days was a turning point for Simon, his lazy habits of beer and biscuits had made him unhappy. "I woke up after my graduation hungover, overweight and wanting to change," he says.

"I started off by setting myself two targets – to cut my calories to 1,500 a day and to start jogging 10k, three times a week. My first major goal was to run in the Glasgow half-marathon." His aspiration to compete in a major event helped him stay motivated. This is an easy way you can keep your weight-loss efforts on track. Head to

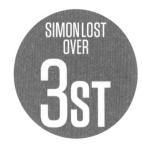

SIMON LOST OVER

3ST

runnersworld.co.uk to find an up-to-date list of all the events in your part of the country.

"After completing the race, I switched to two weekly 16k runs and one 5k run, along with a weights session," says Simon.

KNOCK OUT FAT

With the race over, Simon shifted the focus of his workouts. One of the best ways to keep fat burning on track is to ensure that you're always setting yourself new challenges, that way you won't risk boredom. "I started doing some boxing training," he says. "I would do 5 minutes skipping, 5 minutes bag work and 3 sets of 20 press-ups, interspersed with 1 minute shadow-boxing with 7kg dumb-bells," says Simon.

But not all of Simon's fat burning happened in the gym. "I stopped using the lift at work and changed my route to the office so I'd walk more," he says. Never miss a chance to burn fat, even by standing up to answer your phone at work you'll torch extra calories and it all adds up.

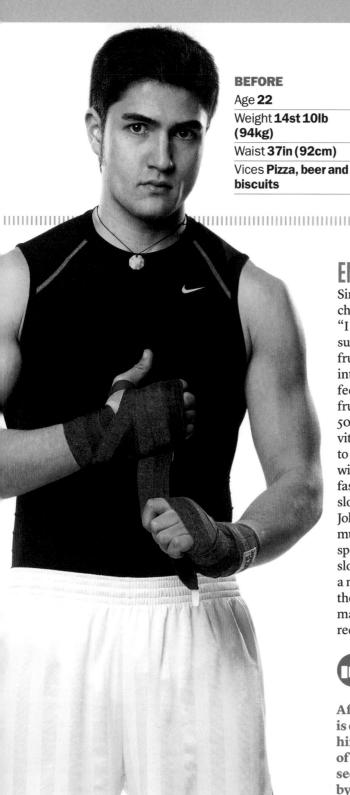

BEFORE		AFTER
Age **22**		Age **22**
Weight **14st 10lb (94kg)**		Weight **11st 3lb (71kg)**
Waist **37in (92cm)**		Waist **30in (75cm)**
Vices **Pizza, beer and biscuits**		Victories **Better sleep, charity fund-raising**

ENTER THE DRAGON

Simon's eating habits also changed from his student diet: "I started eating exotic fruits such as Fuji apples and dragon fruit. The flavours kept me interested and the fibre kept me feeling fuller for longer." Dragon fruit is rich in fibre and provides 50% of your recommended daily vitamin C. Another useful trick is to eat more slowly. Music can help with this. "On a run I listened to fast music, but switched to slower tunes when eating." Johns Hopkins University found music can influence eating speed. Test subjects listening to slow music had three mouthfuls a minute – compared to five by those listening to a fast beat – making digestion easier and reducing fat storage.

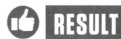 **RESULT**

After losing 3 stone, Simon is continuing to challenge himself with intense intervals of body weight exercises (eg 20 seconds of press-ups followed by 10 seconds rest for 8 sets).

PART

FOUR

MAINTENANCE

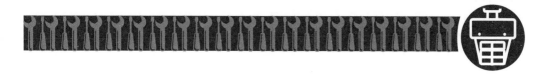

10

THE
SIX-PACK
WORKOUT

YOU'VE BURNT FAT, NOW IT'S
TIME TO REVEAL YOUR ABS

YOU MAY THINK THAT SPORTING A SIX-PACK of abdominal muscles is an impossible dream. We beg to differ. Or maybe sculpting rippling abs just doesn't make your top 10 list of life's priorities. That's fine. You can be fit without looking like Michelangelo's David. But that doesn't mean you can forget about an abdominal workout. It's one of the key commandments of the *Fat Burner's Bible*. Not because abs exercises will melt your gut (they won't), but because you never know when there will be a sale on tinned soup at Tesco. Lifting 24 large tins at once is difficult enough, but without a strong core you run the risk of a strain that could keep you out of action for a long time. Trust us, there are plenty of men who have discovered this the hard way.

YOUR CORE MUSCLES ARE YOUR DEFENCE against the unexpected dangers of modern life. Think about it. Every movement you make originates from your centre of gravity, the core muscles of your torso, which include the abs, the obliques and the pelvis and back muscles. Lift a child. Thank your core muscles, not your biceps. Get out of bed. High-five your abs. Core is key, whether you're sitting, dancing or having sex. And if you want more power in your golf swing, bowling arm or tennis serve, you have to go to the source.

Your core is more than your abs, so before we start conditioning it, let's take a look at the biomechanics of this pivotal area.

1. Rectus Abdominis
Running from your breastbone to your pubic bone, this is the muscle responsible for the six-pack look. It helps flex the spinal column and is active during forward movements, such as crunches. During side-bending motions, these muscles help to stabilise the trunk.

2. External and Internal Obliques
Located on each side of the rectus abdominis, the fibres of these muscles run diagonally across your midsection. The obliques work together to rotate your torso from side to side, allow sideways bending, and contribute to compression of the abdomen.

3. Transverse Abdominis
This deep layer of abdominal muscles wraps around the torso from front to back like a weight belt. It stabilizes the spine, protects the internal organs, and helps with breathing.

4. Hip Flexors
These muscles play a crucial rule in many core exercise movements. They are made up of two groups. One attaches your pelvis to your thighbones, and the other attaches your lower back to your thighbones. Together they are responsible for drawing your legs to your midsection.

Now you know a bit more about the muscles in your core, turn the page for some of the best exercises to work them.

My 6-pack

SIX MOVES THAT WILL GET YOU A SIX-PACK

ONCE YOU HAVE COMPLETED FOUR WEEKS of *The Fat Burner's Bible* workout plan, you should start adding at least one six-pack circuit to your regime each week. It will only take five minutes, but it will help you to look better, feel better and drastically reduce your chances of injury. To keep things interesting, and to keep your muscles guessing, we've included more moves here than you'll need for a circuit. All you need to do is pick four from the following six and then perform 10-20 reps of each with no rest in between. Skipping rest periods will help to give you an excellent fat-burning cardio workout at the same time.

Don't go for more than two weeks without changing the exercises. This will keep your muscles guessing (and growing). It's always best to do your abs circuit at the beginning of your bodyweight or weights workouts and you'll be less likely to blow them off because you are tired or out of time.

TRUNK TWIST

Holding dumbbells, bend your arms and bring the weights close to your belly (**A**). Now slowly twist your torso to the right as far as you can go (**B**). Hold for a couple of seconds, then slowly return to the starting position. Alternate the movements until your you've done 20 repetitions on each side. This will give your obliques a great workout.

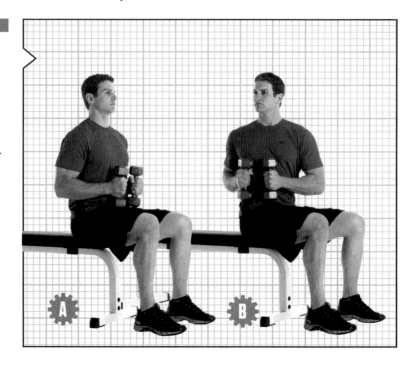

BICYCLE

Lie on your back with your knees bent at 90 degrees and your fingertips lightly touching your ears (**A**). Pump your legs back and forth, bicycle style, while rotating your torso from side to side (**B**). You should try toward the opposite knee on each pump. That'll accentuate your torso rotation. Breathe evenly throughout the exercise. This works your abs and hip flexors.

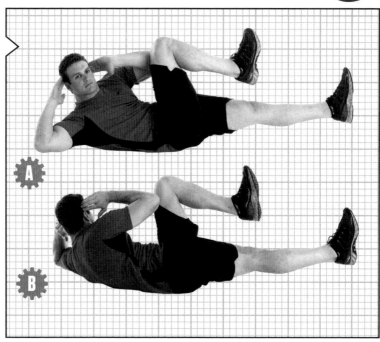

BACK TWIST

This works your transverse abdominis, particularly round your back, for balance. Lie on a Swiss ball as shown. Rest your torso on the ball (**A**). Then raise up and twist your upper body to the right (**B**). Pause for a moment, then lower your torso to the starting position and twist to the left. Pause, then return to the starting position. That's 1 rep. You need to do at least 10.

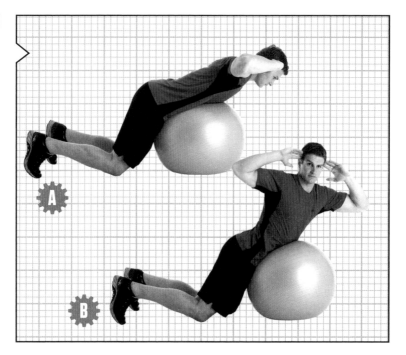

WEIGHTED CRUNCH

Get into the crunch position with your knees bent and feet flat on the floor. Hold either a light medicine ball or a light dumbbell and extend your arms back behind your head (**A**). Now crunch forward, keeping your arms straight (**B**). Do the crunch slowly, and keep your arms straight throughout the exercise. This will help to give your upper abs the best possible workout.

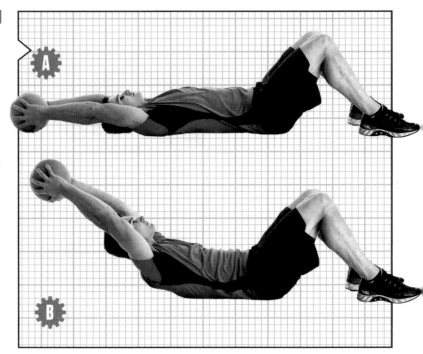

MEDICINE BALL TORSO ROTATION

Kneel down on the floor. Hold a medicine ball or football in front of you. Quickly twist to your right and set the ball down behind your back (**A**). Twist to the left and pick up the ball (**B**). Bring the ball around to your right and set it down again. That's one rep. Repeat until you've done 20. This is great for working your obliques.

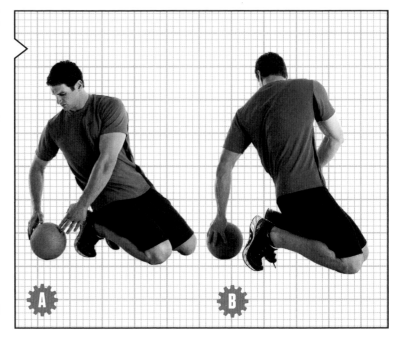

MOTIVATING APPS

Stay on target with a PT in your pocket

NIKE TRAINING CLUB
iPhone, free

This app has a load of built-in workout routines and accompanying videos. Set your fitness level, and it suggests workouts depending on your selection. A great app for beginner gym-goers and those looking for some more workout inspiration.

GYMPACT
iPhone, free

Innovative new app that encourages you to hit the gym with financial incentives. You set yourself gym goals and if you don't go (tracked by GPS) you have to pay a fine. If you do, though, you earn money generated by others' broken pacts. It's ideal if you're finding it difficult to get off the sofa.

HUNDRED PUSHUPS
iPhone, £1.49

Using the in-built accelerometer of your phone, this app measures the amount of press-ups you do in a session, recording your progress over days, weeks and months with graphs and charts. A fantastic app to boost your satisfaction levels as you see yourself progress.

M-TRAIN
iPhone, free

A step-by-step virtual personal trainer that offers fat-burning workouts set to your own music. You select the tunes, it selects the moves that match it – and then you get shredded. It's the next-best thing to having a PT working with you… and complete control of the gym juke box, of course.

SUPERMAN

Lie face down and extend your arms in front of you. Raise your arms and legs off the floor. Hold for 2 seconds, then release and repeat. Your lower back and transverse abdominis will benefit.

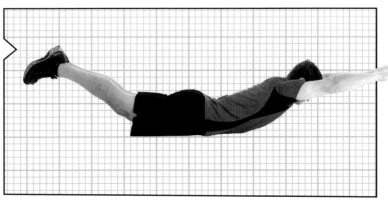

CASE STUDY

John Lamont, from Northern Ireland, showed America the true meaning of 'football', and kicked off his belly in the process

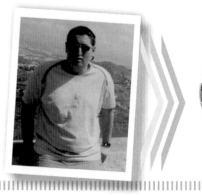

"I COULDN'T BELIEVE HOW BIG I WAS"

John saw himself in a home video at his fattest, most lethargic and unappealing – it was enough to spark his six-stone weight-loss programme.

"I knew I had to make changes. I'd often watch that video later for 'thin-spiration'," he says. Using tools like this can keep you focussed on your weight-loss goals, but you don't have to make a video. A photo of yourself at your fattest can work just as well. Set it as your phone wallpaper so you'll have a reminder of how far you've come.

After a long time out of action, John rediscovered one of his favourite past-times. "I got back into my main love – football – playing twice weekly." In a Copenhagen University study of 14 footballers and 14 joggers, the footballers lost – on average – 7.7lb (3.5kg) of fat and gained 4.4lb (2kg) of muscle over three months. The joggers lost 4.4lb of fat and gained no muscle, so if you've ever enjoyed playing the beautiful game it's time to dust off your boots.

John knew he had to make changes to his lifestyle to get himself back to match fitness. "I eased up on late-night snacks – and the late nights, full stop. As the football progressed and the weight came off I really valued a night's rest." Sleep an extra hour each night to drop a whole stone (6kg) in a year. Michigan University scientist found when sleep replaces idle evening activities you snack less.

BEAT FAT FAST

The exercise didn't stop with football. John started improving his fitness with cardio training: "Music really helped my

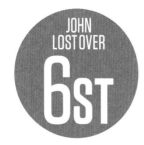

JOHN LOST OVER

6ST

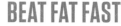

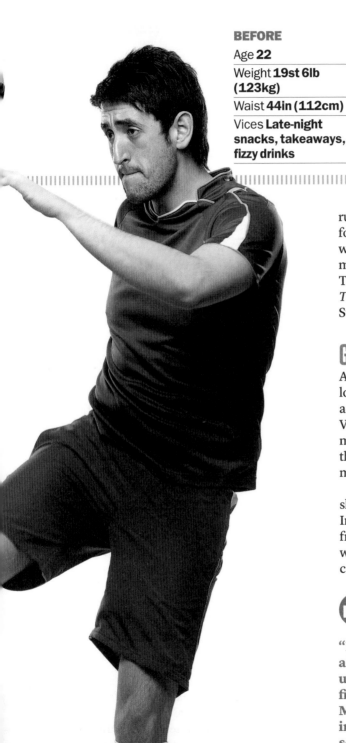

BEFORE		AFTER
Age **22**		Age **24**
Weight **19st 6lb (123kg)**		Weight **13st 4lb (85kg)**
Waist **44in (112cm)**		Waist **34in (86cm)**
Vices **Late-night snacks, takeaways, fizzy drinks**		Victories **Confidence, sports performance, improved social life**

running." St Mary's University found men handle higher workloads when listening to mixes that build in tempo. Try The Rolling Stones' *Sympathy For The Devil* (116 bpm) building to Stereophonics' *Dakota* (148 bpm).

GET SOCIAL

A good way to keep your weight loss on track is to make it a social activity. "I spent a year at West Virginia University," says John. "I made friends with other students through football, and they helped me keep fit and shun TV dinners."

But that didn't mean he also shunned post-match celebrations. Instead John made the switch from beer to vodka and soda, which helped cut out excess calories and carbs.

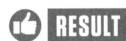 **RESULT**

"I returned home to Ireland a better player – and my university team reached the finals of the All-Ireland Cup. My fortunes with women have improved, too." Now John is scoring on and off the pitch.

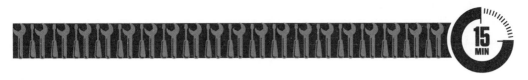

11

DO-ANYWHERE
15-MINUTE
WORKOUTS

> **QUARTER OF AN HOUR IS ALL
> YOU NEED TO STAY IN SHAPE**

HOW MANY TIMES HAVE YOU THOUGHT, "I just don't have time to exercise"? Lack of time is the number one reason people say that they have difficulty sticking with a fitness programme. Time. It's our most precious personal commodity. Other priorities – work, eating, family, socialising, watching YouTube – take precedence over exercise time. But you know that. So, what if working out took just a little bit of time? Say, 15 minutes? Could you find 15 minutes to squeeze in something so vital to your life, so vital to the way you look and feel and the way you perform during the rest of your day? In 24 hours there are 96 individual 15-minute segments – 64, if you subtract the time you spend asleep. That's 64 opportunities to fit exercise into your day.

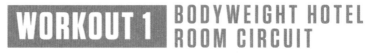

FINDING THE 15 ISN'T HARD. DOING THE 15 – THAT'S THE TOUGH PART.
Taking that first step out of your street clothes and into your shorts. Lacing up your running shoes. Getting moving. All of that is up to you. Nobody is going to take you by the hand. But it helps to have a plan. So here is yours. In this chapter, you'll find 13 different workouts designed to take no longer than 15 minutes. They are brief, but that doesn't mean they are easy. In fact, because you do them so quickly, some of them may have you vomiting in the bushes. But that's okay. Wipe off your shoes. Exercise perfect form, push yourself hard, and you will experience total-body, belly-busting pumps that'll rival most workouts that take an hour or longer. Your 15 minutes starts now.

ANY WEEK, ANY TIME, ANYWHERE

The first two workouts in this section use only your bodyweight (you're getting pretty familiar with this type of workout by now, right?). The third one uses just one piece of equipment: a medicine ball. They're all designed to be extremely versatile so you can slot them into your day whenever you get a moment. First up, the hotel-room circuit, which, of course, you can do just as easily in your own home...

WORKOUT 1 — BODYWEIGHT HOTEL ROOM CIRCUIT

Complete this circuit twice without resting.

EXERCISE	REPS/TIME
PLANK	30 SECONDS IN POSITION 1 30 SECONDS IN POSITION 2
SPLIT SQUAT	10 REPS PER SIDE
T-PRESS-UP	10-20 REPS
STEP-UP	10-20 REPS PER SIDE

TWO-STAGE PLANK

Get into press-up position with your body forming a straight line (A). Hold the pose for 30 seconds while tightening your abs. Next, bend your elbows so that you support your body with your forearms on the floor (B). Hold this position for 30 seconds. This may look easy, but after a few seconds, it really starts to get tough. Keep going until the end of the 30 seconds to start off the workout.

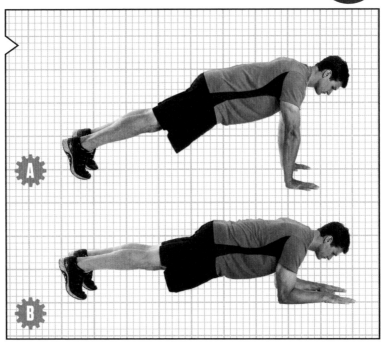

SPLIT SQUAT

Start by standing up straight with your legs roughly hip-width apart. Step forward with your right leg (A). Bend your leg until it forms a 90 degree angle, keeping your right knee facing straight forwards. Lower yourself until your left knee nearly touches the floor (B). Raise yourself back up by extending both legs. Pause, then return to the starting position and repeat for 10 reps each side.

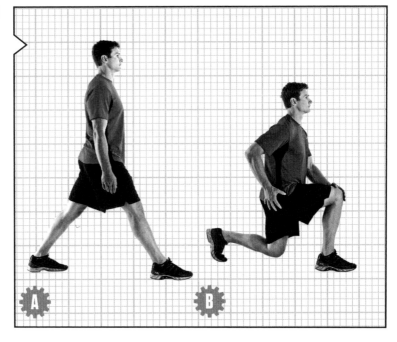

T-PRESS-UP

This one will help your strength and balance. Get into normal press-up position (A). Lower yourself and then push yourself back up (B). When you reach the top position, transfer your weight to your left arm and rotate your body, reaching up with your right arm (C). Hold for 2 seconds. You can make this harder by lifting your leg. Return to the starting position and repeat on the other side with your left arm raised. Perform 10 to 20 repetitions.

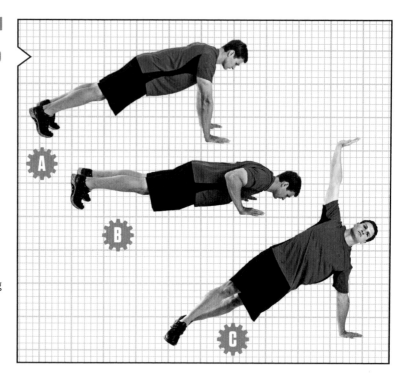

STEP-UP

Find a staircase and stand facing it. Place your right foot on the bottom step (A). Using only your right leg, push yourself up until you can straighten that leg, then lift your left knee as shown (B). Slowly lower yourself, keeping your right foot on the step. Lower your left leg to return to the starting position. Repeat 10-20 times. Then place your left foot on the step to repeat the exercise on the other side.

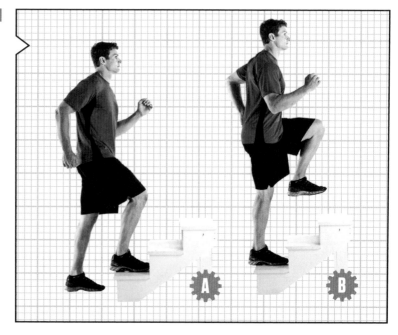

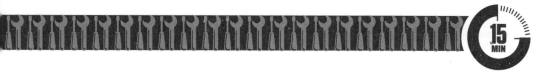

WORKOUT 2 QUICK STEPS

This workout combines cardiovascular drills with strength exercises to build muscle and burn calories. All you need is a staircase or a bench. Alternate between the sprinter's step drill and the elevated-feet press-up for 2 sets before moving onto the upper-body shuttle.

EXERCISE	REPS/TIME
SPRINTER'S STEP DRILL	30 SECONDS
ELEVATED PRESS-UP	10-15 REPS
SPRINTER'S STEP DRILL	30 SECONDS
ELEVATED PRESS-UP	10-15 REPS
UPPER-BODY SHUTTLE	30-60 SECONDS

SPRINTER'S STEP DRILL

Stand facing a step or bench with your right foot on the step and your right knee bent (A). Rapidly alternate your feet on and off the step so you're sprinting on the step (B). Drive your knees up and pump your arms as if you were sprinting. Continue for 30 seconds. This drill is designed to get your blood pumping and your heart rate up. Great for burning calories and shedding pounds.

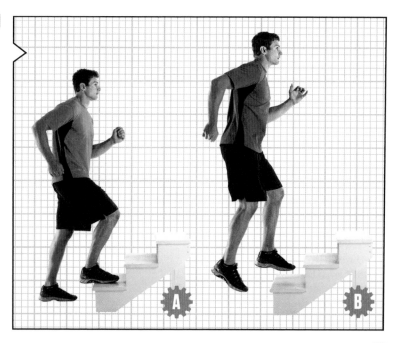

ELEVATED PRESS-UP

A harder version of the classic press-up. Get into the usual position but this time with your feet on a step. Your stairs at home should be ideal. Face away from them with the balls of your feet on the bottom step (A). Brace your abs and keep your back flat. Bend your elbows and lower yourself until your chest is a couple of inches off the floor (B). Pause, then push yourself back up. Do 10-15 reps.

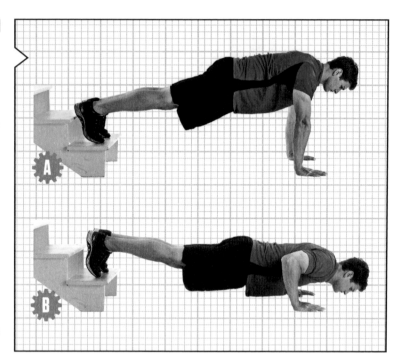

UPPER-BODY SHUTTLE

Turn around and face the stairs, still in a press-up position, with your fingertips just in front of the bottom step (A). Lift one hand onto the step (B), then bring up your other hand (C). Return your first hand to the floor, then the second. Walk your hands up and down this way for 30-60 seconds. Go as fast as you can to give a real boost to this move's calorie-burning effects.

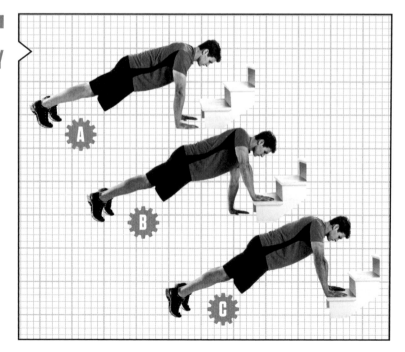

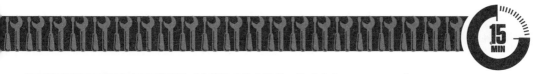

WORKOUT 3 — MEDICINE-BALL LADDER

15 MIN

This gruelling four-drill circuit incinerates belly fat in less time than it takes to make your supper – in fact you could do it while it's in the oven. Incorporating a medicine ball adds interest, difficulty, and an upper-body element. Do each of the exercises for 30 seconds, then rest for 1 minute. Repeat the circuit, this time performing each move for 45 seconds. Rest for 90 seconds, then repeat once more, doing each move for 60 seconds.

EXERCISE	REPS/TIME
SIDE SHUFFLE	30 SECONDS
OVERHEAD LUNGE WALK	30 SECONDS
MEDICINE BALL 180	30 SECONDS
PRESS-UP SHUTTLE	30 SECONDS
REST	1 MINUTE
SIDE SHUFFLE	45 SECONDS
OVERHEAD LUNGE WALK	45 SECONDS
MEDICINE BALL 180	45 SECONDS
PRESS-UP SHUTTLE	45 SECONDS
REST	90 SECONDS
SIDE SHUFFLE	60 SECONDS
OVERHEAD LUNGE WALK	60 SECONDS
MEDICINE BALL 180	60 SECONDS
PRESS-UP SHUTTLE	60 SECONDS

GYM TIP

Mix it up. Never do the same workout for more than four weeks at a time. If you do, your body will get used to the moves and your muscle gain and fat loss will start to plateau.

SIDE SHUFFLE

Stand about 5 feet away from a wall, facing towards it. Lean forward slightly and hold a medicine ball at your chest (A). Throw the ball at the wall 3-5 feet to your right and at eye level (B). As the ball bounces off the wall, shuffle sideways and catch it on a bounce before firing it back to your left (C). This drill helps to improve co-ordination as well as building upper-body strength and burning fat.

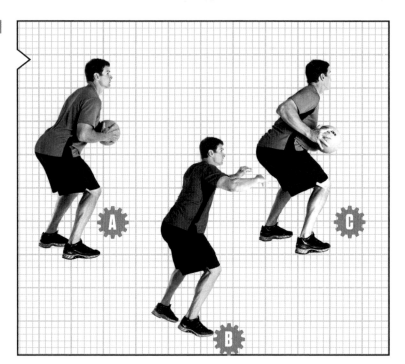

OVERHEAD LUNGE WALK

Stand by holding a medicine ball over your head at arm's length (A). Keeping your arms straight throughout the move, take a large step forward until both knees are bent 90 degrees and your back knee is an inch or two off the floor (B). Then stride forward with the opposite leg (C), and keep alternating legs (D). This tough routine will build the large muscles in your legs which will aid fat-burning.

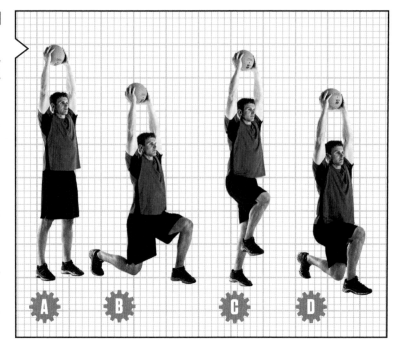

MEDICINE BALL 180

Stand about 5 feet away from a wall so that the right side of your body is facing it. Hold a medicine ball in front of your chest. Rotate your torso away from the wall (A), then rotate forcefully toward the wall, throwing the ball slightly behind you (B). Turn around and shuffle over to catch the ball on a bounce (C), then repeat the move in the opposite direction (D). Continue for the specified number of seconds.

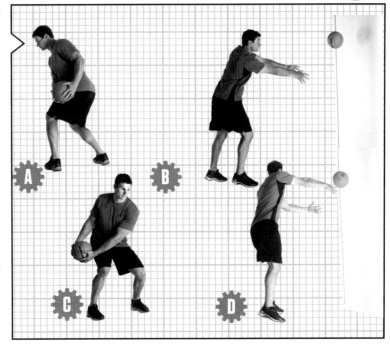

PRESS-UP SHUTTLE

Assume the classic press-up position, but instead of placing both hands on the floor, place your right hand on a medicine ball (A). Bend your arms slowly to lower your body toward the floor (B). Push yourself up, then transfer your left hand to the medicine ball (C). Next, move your right hand to the floor (D) to perform a pushup (E). Repeat for the specified number of seconds and then rest.

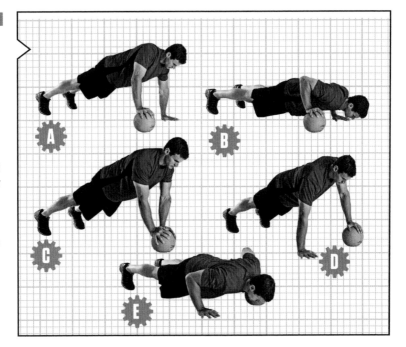

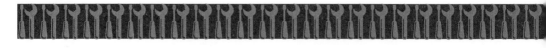

FAST, FAT-BURNING, CARDIO INTERVALS

Not sure you've got time for three cardio workouts a week? Well, with these 15 minute sessions you have. These intervals will burn just as much fat as a steady 45-minute jog in the park, in a third of the time. So, why not make these the rule, and longer workouts the exception? First up, the 'original' intervals, Fartlek...

WORKOUT 4 STEP-DOWN FARTLEK

Fartlek is Swedish for 'speed play,' meaning you accelerate and slow down according to how you feel. Basically you sprint as hard as you can for as long as you can before slowing down to catch your breath. Then repeat. Or choose two points ahead of you, a telephone pole, for example, and a postbox 50-100 metres ahead. You sprint between them before slowing down to recover and then repeating with another set of landmarks. In a step-down fartlek, you remove the 'choice' element and follow a structure. The intervals become harder, mimicking the end of a race.

EXERCISE	REPS/TIME
RUN AT 60% EFFORT	2.5 MINUTES
RUN AT 40% EFFORT	2.5 MINUTES
RUN AT 70% EFFORT	2 MINUTES
RUN AT 40% EFFORT	2 MINUTES
RUN AT 80% EFFORT	1.5 MINUTES
RUN AT 40% EFFORT	1.5 MINUTES
RUN AT 90% EFFORT	1 MINUTE
RUN AT 40% EFFORT	2 MINUTES

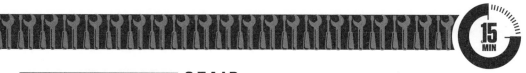

WORKOUT 5 — STAIR SPRINTS

Find a large flight of stairs at a town hall, footbridge or steep street

EXERCISE	REPS/TIME
SPRINT TO TOP OF STAIRS, WALK BACK DOWN	10 REPS
REST	60 SECONDS
SPRINT TO TOP OF STAIRS, WALK BACK DOWN	10 REPS
REST	60 SECONDS
SPRINT UP FOUR STEPS, JOG BACK DOWN	
SPRINT UP FIVE STEPS, JOG BACK DOWN	
REPEAT UNTIL YOU REACH TO TOP OF THE STEPS	

WORKOUT 6 — ROWING FAT-BURNER

You can burn 40 to 50 percent more fat when rowing than when cycling because rowing machines require equal effort from your upper and lower body.

EXERCISE	REPS/TIME
EASY ROWING WARM-UP	5 MINUTES
POWER STROKES (MAXIMUM EFFORT)	10 REPS
HALF EFFORT	60 SECONDS
POWER STROKES	15 REPS
HALF EFFORT	60 SECONDS
POWER STROKES	20 REPS
EASY ROWING	60 SECONDS
REPEAT CYCLE WITHOUT WARM-UP FOR 10 MINUTES	

EASY LIFESTYLE TWEAK

Get into crosswords. Often we snack when we're bored, particularly when waiting around in stations or airports. Instead of grabbing a burger, grab a newspaper and do the crossword. It will keep your mind and hands occupied.

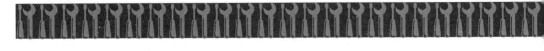

WORKOUT 7 — KNEE-SAVING ELLIPTICAL INTERVAL

This workout it specifically designed for the elliptical machine. To boost the cardiovascular benefits and burn more calories, don't hold the machine, pump your arms as if you were running.

EXERCISE	REPS/TIME
WARM-UP	5 MINUTES
HIGH RESISTANCE AT 80% EFFORT	2 MINUTES
LOW-RESISTANCE AT 80% EFFORT	2 MINUTES
HIGH RESISTANCE AT 80% EFFORT	2 MINUTES
LOW-RESISTANCE AT 80% EFFORT	2 MINUTES

WORKOUT 8 — UP-THE-INCLINE TREADMILL INTERVAL

Intervals doesn't always mean changing speed. You can do it with incline, too. Because treadmills are powered, they're slightly easier than running on the road. However, research shows that an incline of 1 percent mimics the effort of outdoor running more closely. So that's where this workout starts...

GYM TIP

Research conducted at the University of New South Wales, Australia found that sprinting on a bike for 8 seconds followed by 12 seconds of recovery burned much more fat over 40 minutes than cycling at one speed. This can be applied to any cardio exercise, so there's no excuse to take it easy.

EXERCISE	REPS/TIME
JOG AT 60% EFFORT, 1% INCLINE	2 MINUTES
JOG AT THE SAME SPEED, 4% INCLINE	2 MINUTES
SAME SPEED, 6% INCLINE	2 MINUTES
SAME SPEED, 8% INCLINE	2 MINUTES
SAME SPEED 10% INCLINE	2 MINUTES
REDUCE INCLINE BY 1%	EVERY 30 SECONDS

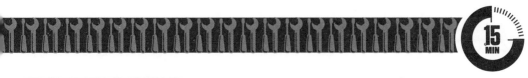

WORKOUT 9 — EASY RUNNING INTERVAL OUTDOORS

The following workout is an excellent step toward building the stamina for high-intensity interval training.

EXERCISE	REPS/TIME
WARM-UP	5 MINUTES
SPRINT	30 SECONDS
RECOVERY	90 SECONDS
REPEAT THE SPRINTS AND RECOVERIES THREE MORE TIMES	

WORKOUT 10 — TOUGH RUNNING INTERVAL OUTDOORS

This is a really intense fat-burner. The time of each sprint decreases as the intensity decreases and you only get 30 seconds recovery after each one.

EXERCISE	REPS/TIME
WARM-UP	5 MINUTES
SPRINT (70% EFFORT)	30 SECONDS
SPRINT (75% EFFORT)	25 SECONDS
SPRINT (80% EFFORT)	25 SECONDS
SPRINT (85% EFFORT)	20 SECONDS
SPRINT (90% EFFORT)	20 SECONDS
SPRINT (95% EFFORT)	15 SECONDS
SPRINT (100% EFFORT)	10 SECONDS
COOL-DOWN	5 MINUTES
RECOVER FROM EACH SPRINT WITH 30 SECONDS JOG AT 60% EFFORT	

EASY LIFESTYLE TWEAK

Take the stairs over the lift whenever possible. Not only will you build a fat-burning workout into your day, but a survey published in the *Canadian Medical Association Journal* found you'll save time. In the study it took an average of 13 seconds to go one floor by stairs, compared to 37 seconds in a lift (most of that time spent waiting).

ROPE TRICKS

SKIPPING WILL HELP YOU SKIP BIG MEALS

A skipping rope is one of the cheapest yet most effective pieces of exercise equipment. If you don't have one, put down this book and buy one. Just 10 minutes of skipping can burn the same amount of calories as 30 minutes of running. The dynamic movements will enhance your performance in virtually any sport. Plus, when you get good enough to do those front crosses and single side swings, you'll look like a prizefighter – featherweight, of course.

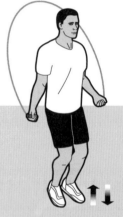

THE BASIC MOVE
Keep your weight on the balls of your feet. Bend your knees slightly. The trick is to keep your jumps shallow; don't jump more than an inch. Keep your body upright and elbows at your sides. Make small circles with your wrists. The jump comes from the movement of your ankles, calves, knees, and hips. Point your toes downward as you lift off. Land softly by spreading the impact through your ankles, knees, and hips. Don't think too hard. Just keep your heels from touching the ground.

SIDE-TO-SIDE
Keeping your feet together, jump alternately a few inches from left to right. Keep on your toes. This style involves more muscles in lateral movement, including your core, obliques and hip flexors. More calories are burned this way than basic skipping and it will improve your footwork on the football field.

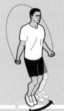

ALTERNATE HIGH JUMPS
Just like the regular skip, but while jumping on one foot, bring your other knee up to your chest then back down before the rope comes around. Alternate with legs. Start off slowly to get used to it then turn up the tempo. High knee skips are good for working your abdominals and for improving leg strength.

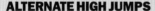

CRISS-CROSS
You need to jump as normal but begin crossing your arms as the rope goes over your head. By the time you jump your hands should be at your pockets, making a loop big enough to jump through. As the rope comes back over your head again, uncross your arms. This gives your upper body a workout along with your legs.

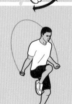

ADVANCED INTERVALS
Pack a skipping rope in your suitcase on your next business trip. The following 15-minute drill will give you an unparalleled total-body workout, anywhere.

● Warm up with 3 minutes of easy skipping.
● Increase your speed to 80 percent of your maximum effort for 30 seconds.
● Skip easily for 60 seconds.
● Do high-knee skips for 30 seconds.
● Skip easily for 60 seconds.
● Continue this pattern for two more cycles.
● For the last 3 minutes, alternate between skipping as fast as you can for 60 seconds and skipping easily for 60 seconds

SUPER-QUICK WEIGHTS WORKOUTS

Adding some weight to your workouts is the fastest way to make them more effective. Always pick dumbbells heavy enough to challenge you and have you failing on your final set, and you'll fat-burning will be well and truly supercharged.

WORKOUT 11 — WEIGHTED PUSH-PULLS

Do the sets and reps as outlined below. Rest 30 seconds between sets.

EXERCISE	REPS/SETS
BULGARIAN SPLIT SQUAT PRESS	8-10 x 3
SQUAT PRESS	8-10 x 3
SINGLE-ARM PRESS ON SWISS BALL	8-10 x 3
BENT-OVER ROW AND ROMANIAN DEADLIFT	8-10 x 3

BULGARIAN SPLIT-SQUAT PRESS

Bend your right knee and place your right foot on a bench behind you with dumbbells at your shoulders (A). As you descend into a squat, press the dumbbells overhead (B). As you straighten your left leg, bring the weights back to your shoulders. Do 8-10 reps, then switch legs.

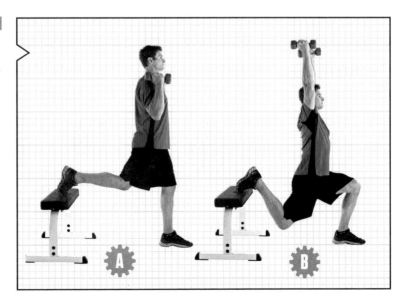

SQUAT PRESS

Stand with feet roughly shoulder-width apart and hold dumbbells at your shoulders, with your palms facing each other (**A**). Descend slowly into into a deep squat, keeping your back straight, but with a natural arch at all times (**B**). Drive the weights overhead as you rise from the bottom of the squat (**C**). As a whole-body workout, it's hard to find anything more complete than this. Do 8-10 reps.

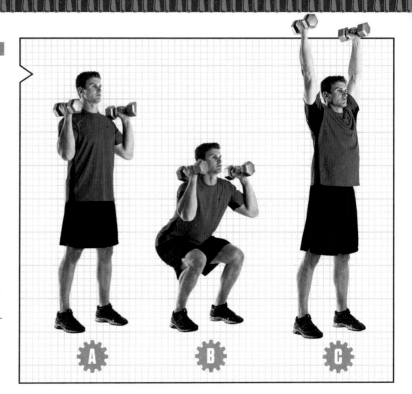

BENT-OVER ROW AND ROMANIAN DEADLIFT

Stand with your feet shoulder-width apart, holding a barbell (**A**). Bend at the waist until your lower back is flat (**B**); bend your knees slightly. Row the weight up until your lower rib cage (**C**). Lower the bar until your arms are completely extended (**D**). Return to the starting position (**E**). Do 8-10 reps.

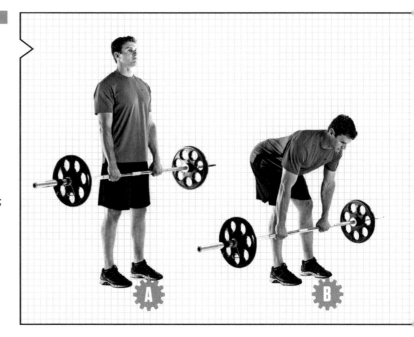

SINGLE-ARM PRESS ON SWISS BALL

Lie with your upper back on a Swiss ball and hold a dumbbell in your left hand at your chest, with your palm facing your feet (A). Press the weight slowly up, attempting to keep the rest of your body as still as possible (B). Do 8-10 reps, then transfer the dumbbell to your right hand and repeat the same number of reps. This is an excellent workout for your core, arms and chest.

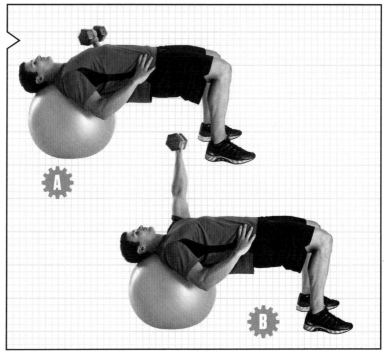

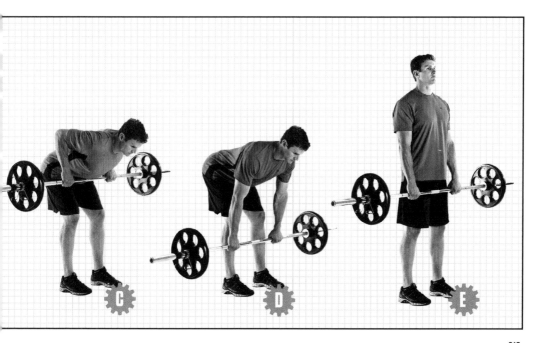

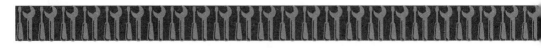

WORKOUT 12 — STOP-AND-GO SUPERSETS

The stop-and-go is a terrific plateau-busting workout. It works by adding two-second pauses into basic moves, which you've probably already mastered. By interrupting momentum at various power points, you recruit more muscle fibres, making each rep a lot tougher. Consequently you'll probably need to switch to a significantly lighter weight than you usually pick up for these moves. This may feel like a step back, but trust us, the results are worth it. You're guaranteed more calories burned and more strength at your weak spots.

To make this workout even more effective the exercises are in supersets. As you'll remember, if you tackled them on as part of the Bodyweight plan earlier in this book, supersets are paired exercises with no rest in between. They get your heart pumping faster than regular weights workouts, and so are excellent for fat burning.

Do the exercises as outlined in the table below. First up is press-ups and split squats with no rest between exercises. Then rest for 30 seconds and repeat the superset. Next, do the dumbbell row and the sumo squat as another superset. Again, repeat this superset. So by the end of the workout you'll have done eight sets in four supersets. Good luck.

EASY LIFESTYLE TWEAK

Always try to get 6-8 hours sleep a night. A study at the University of Chicago found that when you are sleep deprived your body misinterprets your lack of energy as being cause by a lack of fuel and so ramps up your hunger levels.

EXERCISE	REPS OR TIME
Superset 1	
STOP-AND-GO PRESS-UP	8 REPS
STOP-AND-GO SPLIT SQUAT	8 REPS
REST	30 SECONDS
Superset 2	
STOP-AND-GO INCLINE ROW	10 REPS
STOP-AND-GO SUMO SQUAT	10 REPS

WORKOUT 12 SUPERSET 1

STOP-AND-GO PRESS-UP

Assume a press-up position (A). Brace your core and lower your chest to the floor (B). When you're halfway down, pause for 2 seconds before continuing. Then, when your chest is 2 inches from the floor, pause again for 2 seconds before pushing halfway back up. Hold for 2 more seconds, then straighten your arms. Do 8 reps.

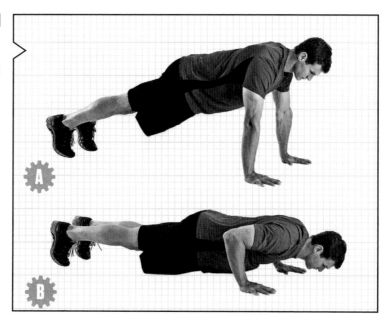

STOP-AND-GO SPLIT SQUAT

Stand with one foot on a step roughly 3ft (1m) in front of you (A). Rise on the ball of your back foot, then bend at the knees (B). When you're halfway down, pause for 2 seconds. Pause again when your back knee is just off the floor. Push halfway up, pause again for 2 seconds, and return to the starting position. Do 8 reps with each leg.

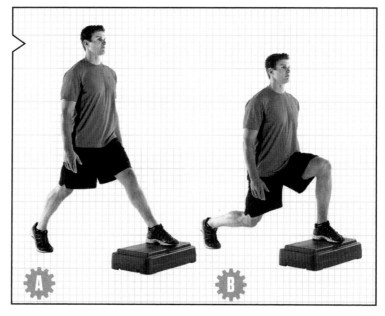

WORKOUT 12 SUPERSET 2

STOP-AND-GO INCLINE ROW

Holding dumbbells, lie facedown on a bench set at 45 degrees (A). Pull the dumbbells up towards you (B). When your upper arms align with your torso, pause 2 seconds before continuing until the weights are at your sides. Hold for two more seconds, then lower halfway and pause again. Return to the starting position. Do 10 reps.

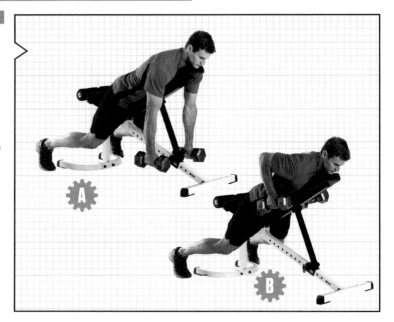

STOP-AND-GO SUMO SQUAT

Stand holding a barbell across your shoulders, feet wide apart with toes turned out (A). (You can also do this without weights). Bend your knees. Halfway down, pause 2 seconds before continuing until your thighs are parallel to the floor (B). Pause two beats, then press halfway up and pause again. Do 10 reps and the rest.

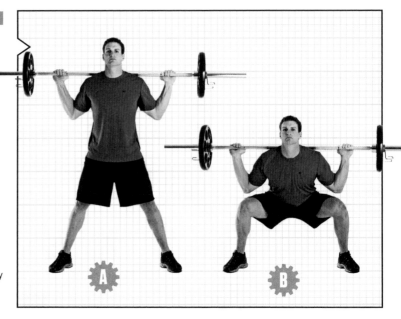

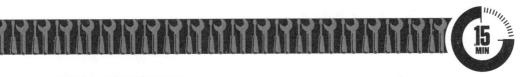

WORKOUT 13 — THE TWO-SET CLASSIC

This workout compiles many of the classic moves you have already learned in previous workouts. You need to do two sets of each, resting for 30 seconds between sets. There's a lot to fit in in 15 minutes, but if you organise your equipment first and are strict about timings, you should be able to do it.

SQUAT

SET 1	8-12 REPS
SET 2	6-8 REPS

FORWARD LUNGE

SET 1	8-12 REPS
SET 2	6-8 REPS

DUMBBELL BENCH PRESS

SET 1	8-12 REPS
SET 2	6-8 REPS

BENT-OVER-ROW

SET 1	8-12 REPS
SET 2	6-8 REPS

SEATED DUMBBELL SHOULDER PRESS

SET 1	8-12 REPS
SET 2	6-8 REPS

BICEP CURL

SET 1	8-12 REPS
SET 2	6-8 REPS

CRUNCH

SET 1	TO FAILURE

EASY LIFESTYLE TWEAK

A study conducted at University College in London found ambitious weight-loss goals are the most effective. But the American Council on Exercise found attainability is important to maintain motivation. The best solution? Set both short and long-term fat-burning goals.

CASE STUDY

Robb Cayford from Bishop's Stortford hit an emotional low, took one look at the man in the mirror and then ran for his life

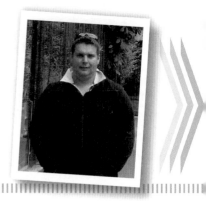

"BEING FAT RUINED MY LOVE LIFE"

I took some shock treatment to kick-start Robb's weight loss. "I split up with my girlfriend and realised I'd have to lose weight if I was ever to date again. I saw a photo of myself at 20st, and felt really down. I decided there and then that I needed to fight back.

"I started jogging, and invested in good shoes to help me view it as a new habit rather than just a fad." Robb was told to always buy trainers in the late afternoon. "Feet get bigger during the day," says podiatrist Sonal Patel. Try Nike's bespoke 'iD' service (nikeid.nike.com) for a good fit.

ROBB LOST OVER
6ST

"I entered as many races as I could, so I was constantly challenging myself. I also took up weekly five-a-side football," says Robb. A University of Copenhagen study found a game of five-a-side burns up to 800 calories an hour. Competition and challenges are great ways to motivate yourself to exercise, and make your training fun.

FOOD FOR THOUGHT

Robb works as a teacher and stumbled across a useful weight-loss technique in the school canteen. "I'd fill my plate with veg," says Robb. Penn State University research found people eat a consistent weight of food. So swapping pasta for the same volume of veg means you lose weight without snacking.

"Chocolate went from daily essential to one-off treat. I ate healthy replacements instead." An easy way to ensure you do this is, suggests nutritionist Amanda Ursell, is to put dried fruit where you'd normally store sweet things (like in a biscuit tin).

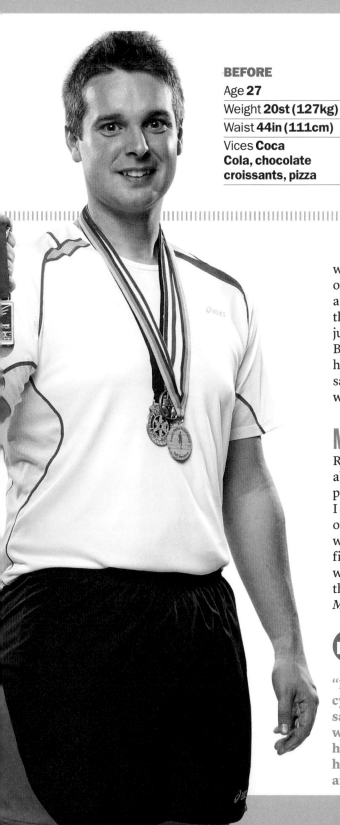

BEFORE	AFTER
Age **27**	Age **29**
Weight **20st (127kg)**	Weight **13.5st (85kg)**
Waist **44in (111cm)**	Waist **33in (84cm)**
Vices **Coca Cola, chocolate croissants, pizza**	Victories **Energy, rediscovered sports, extra confidence**

"Another food swap I made was to go for mixed nuts instead of crisps," says Robb. This is a good idea, because, even though nuts are quite calorific, just a few almonds, pistachios or Brazils each day (nuts that are high in unsaturated fats) will satiate your hunger without widening your waist.

MONEY FOR NOTHING

Robb was so confident in his ability to shift his weight, he even put money on it. "At a wedding, I dressed in the same suit as the other ushers and won a £100 bet with someone who said I'd never fit into it." Financial incentives will help you lose weight, reports the *Journal of the American Medical Association.*

 RESULT

"I hit a plateau at 15½st, but cycling got me through it," says Robb. His dedication to weight loss helped him regain his lost confidence and started him on the road to a new life, and a new love.

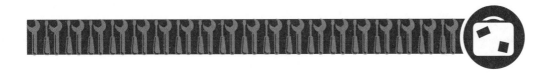

THE ART OF
TRAVELLING
LIGHT

A PLAN TO KEEP WEIGHT OFF WHILE YOU'RE AWAY

WELCOME TO THE FLIGHT OF YOUR DREAMS. You only have to be at the airport an hour before your flight. There's no body search at the security check, and you are free to leave your shoes on. The plane isn't crowded. The seats are leather and roomy. The person sitting next to you is attractive, friendly and interesting. Your bags arrive at your destination at the same time as you. And you won't put on 5 pounds by the time you get back home.

Now wake up. Bring your seat-back and tray table up and put away all unapproved electronic devices. The reality of travel, whether it's for business or pleasure, is that it can easily knock you out of your fitness routine and botch up your best intentions to eat healthily. The moment you get on a plane its easy to grant yourself a licence to eat (and drink) whatever you like.

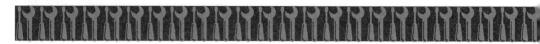

HOLIDAYS ARE AN ESSENTIAL PART OF WINDING DOWN, while business trips are non-negotiable, you can't realistically skip either. But you can stop them from destroying all the hard work you've put in burning fat. There are right ways to travel to minimise the toll on your body, and there are wrong ways. "The problem with holidays and business trips is that people turn them into special events that allow them to break sound nutrition rules," says Susan Bowerman, a dietitian and assistant director for the UCLA Center for Human Nutrition.

Isn't that true? You eat the salted nuts. Drink a beer. Then, why not a little wine with dinner? And surely it would be rude to skip the cheese and the extra glass of wine, seeing as it was so kindly offered... and included in the price of your flight... A little later there's some ice cream and a bit of cognac while watching the movies. Then, before you know it, it's time for breakfast! Bloody Mary anyone?

By the time you arrive you're bleary eyed and covered in crumbs. So, you grab a double espresso. Then, if you're on business there'll be more coffee at every meeting. And tasty little pastries. And, whether its business or pleasure it's easy to slip into a habit of having big lunches with wine. And dinners in the evening, with more wine. Oh, and after-dinner cocktails.

But with a little forward thinking, your next trip doesn't have to be like this. The unhealthy way is the easy way, particularly on flights. It's all laid on for you so you don't have to think. But if you take a step back and actually plan a little, you can curb all the damaging effects on your waistline. Try having a workout first thing before your flight, then you'll be more likely to sleep on the plane. Also, eat before you board or if you have to wait for a connecting flight, that way you'll be in control of what's going in your mouth, rather than leaving yourself at the mercy of the airline galley. Pack snacks for the flight as well. Unsalted nuts are good, bananas are even better as their potassium helps aid restful sleep. With any luck you'll snooze right through temptation (and the terrible in-flight film) and arrive at your destination refreshed and ready to make a good impression with your business associates, or just to explore the local area instead of collapsing in your hotel.

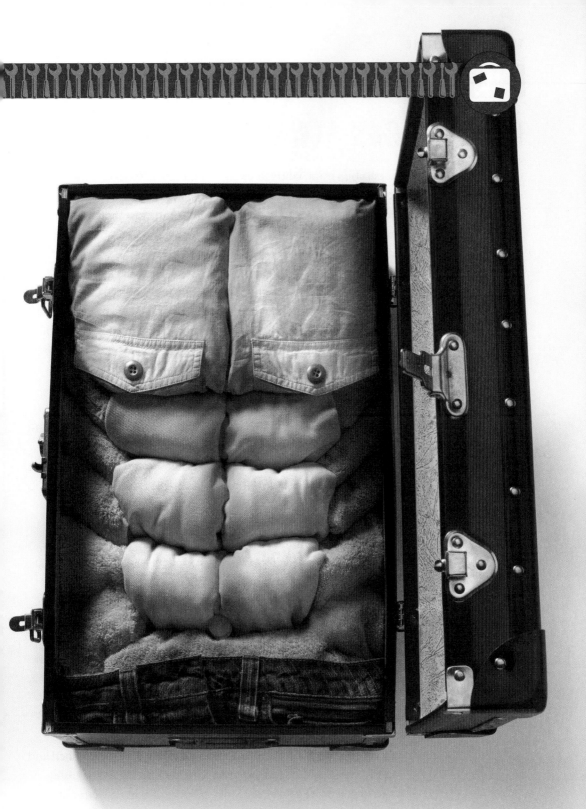

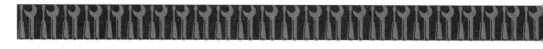

HOW YOU CAN ALWAYS TRAVEL LIGHTER

Preparation is the key to keeping foreign travel from derailing your fat burning – even if you're only staying overnight in Paris. Use these tips to make your getaway an opportunity to leave some extra baggage behind, not to pick up more.

Drink Water On The Way To The Airport

Then sip some more after you make it through check-in. Flying can dehydrate you easily. And cravings are often nothing more than an indication that you are thirsty, not hungry. Have around 100ml of water for every hour that you're in the air.

Be Wary Of Freebies

Don't tempt yourself with the free drinks and salted snacks. Instead, pack carrot sticks, hard-boiled eggs, fruit and slices of ham or turkey to eat while waiting for your flight.

Pack Your Own Peanuts

Better yet, pack unsalted raw almonds. Rich in protein, they'll fill you up and won't make you thirsty.

Always Pack Your Gym Kit

So long as you've got your trainers, shorts and a T-shirt, you can get some exercise done.

Go For A Run When You Arrive

The best way to reset your internal clock on an overnight flight is to get out into the sunshine as soon as you arrive. If it's too early for check-in, drop your bags at the hotel, change into running gear in the hotel gym, and hit the pavement. Exercise is a terrific way to wake up and improve your mood, and running is a great opportunity to soak up some local colour while soaking in some natural light. Ask the concierge to map out a good running route so you won't get lost.

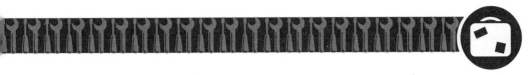

Use Your Bodyweight

Don't forget to use *The Fat Burner's Bible* workouts on your trip. If your hotel doesn't have a gym you can always do a bodyweight routine in your room. You could even try running up and down the hotel's stairs. You're likely to get them all to yourself and it's a great way of doing interval training without needing a treadmill.

Soak Up Healthy Culture

If you're visiting Cornwall, take a surfing lesson; in Holland try cycling; and in Scotland, hike or even ski. On business your hotel concierge can prearrange activities to match your schedule. If you're at leisure, well, just pick your ideal time and get booked in.

Make The Minibar Out-Of-Bounds

The hotel room minibar is an expensive way to gain pounds. When you arrive at the hotel make a promise to yourself not to touch it. Don't even open it. It might even be possible to have it locked, if you feel the temptation of an £8 Toblerone will be too much.

Make It A Date

Prescheduling a fitness date is one of the best ways to guarantee that you won't stop exercising on the road, so invite whoever you are travelling with for a game of tennis, or a run . If you are on business and alone it can be a great way to meet new people and you can use the power of the internet to track them down. Websites like socialgolfer.co.uk and runnersworld.co.uk provide excellent forums for hooking up with like-minded individuals and finding competitions and races, wherever you happen to be in the world.

Carry Supplies

It can be tough to find a protein shake when you're driving through the Dordogne. So carry some with you and zip-top bags of premeasured powder. It will ensure you are only a glass of water away from well-balanced nutrition. On the downside, you may have a bit of explaining to do before you can clear customs...

GYM TIP

If you can, schedule your workout for the morning. A study at the Mayo Clinic in the US found that this is ideal for fat-burning as you have more hours awake afterwards to reap the metabolism-boosting benefits.

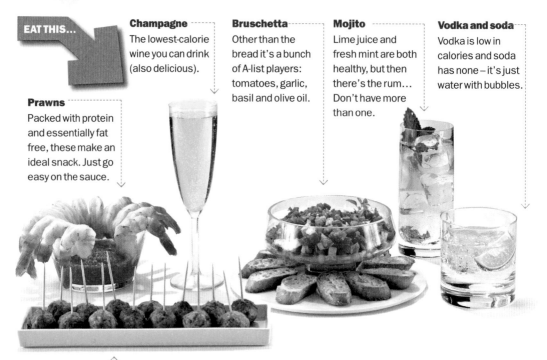

EAT THIS...

Champagne
The lowest-calorie wine you can drink (also delicious).

Bruschetta
Other than the bread it's a bunch of A-list players: tomatoes, garlic, basil and olive oil.

Mojito
Lime juice and fresh mint are both healthy, but then there's the rum... Don't have more than one.

Vodka and soda
Vodka is low in calories and soda has none – it's just water with bubbles.

Prawns
Packed with protein and essentially fat free, these make an ideal snack. Just go easy on the sauce.

Meatballs
These protein-based bites will fill you up fast, saving you from senseless snacking later on.

SURVIVE THE BUFFET

Your toughest obstacle on any trip, business or pleasure, is the all-inclusive buffet. It's full of delicious morsels, fried and sauce-laden. And it's free, which makes it even more tempting. Here are some tricks to keep you from blowing your belly.

Drink A Glass Of Tomato Juice

The pulpy liquid has bulk so will give your stomach some volume to take the edge off your appetite.

Practice Stealth Drinking

Drink a glass of ice water between beer, wine or cocktails. It'll effectively cut your alcohol and calorie intake in half. Or fake it. Order a diet ginger ale in a scotch glass with lemon. No one will know you're not drinking booze and so you won't have to resist peer pressure to indulge.

Gin and tonic
It looks light, but tonic is actually packed with sugar so avoid or go slimline.

Margarita
Often made with sugar-heavy fruit juice. Insist on fresh limes for a healthier hit.

Spinach artichoke dip
Yes, it's got vegetables in. But it's also go cream cheese, double cream, Parmesan and mozzarella. Approach with caution.

Corona
Even lighter tasting beers aren't going to make you feel any lighter

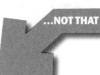

...NOT THAT

Crab cakes
Crab is great. But when its mixed with mayo, rolled in breadcrumbs and fried, it's not really that good any more

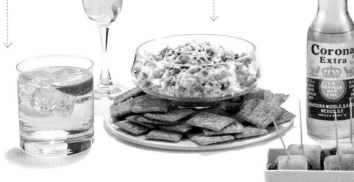

Sausage rolls
The meat is processed but it's the buttery pastry that really ups the calorie count

Take A Small Plate

A study in the *Journal of Consumer Research* found when a variety of foods are offered, such as at a buffet, people eat 43 percent more. So, instead of grabbing the large main-course plate, use the dessert plate and only have two items on it at a time. You'll eat slower, allowing time for feelings of satiety signals to reach your brain.

Make A Buffet-Tray Hit List

Always eat from the vegetable tray first. The high-water-volume, high-fibre fare will fill you up without delivering a lot of calories. Pass by the bread, chips, sauce-laden pastas, and anything fried.

Be The Life And Soul

Focus on the social aspect of the party rather than the eating. Set a goal to talk to seven new people. If you have a mission, you'll be less likely to munch mindlessly.

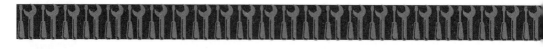

EATING WELL WHEN YOU'RE ON THE ROAD

When you can't prepare your own meals, you give up a lot of control to the restaurant that serves you. So the best thing you can do is control massive portion sizes by leaving food on your plate. We throw nutrition to the wind and ignore portion size when we travel. You need to fight that part of human nature. Here are some other general tips, plus some smart meal choices to help you eat well:

Drink Before You Eat

Make sure you drink lots of water during the day. It'll make you feel fuller so you won't eat as much. Don't wait until mealtime to do this, because fluids dilute digestive enzymes and can hamper absorption of vital nutrients, which are key to efficient energy metabolism. To curb your appetite before a meal, guzzle a couple of glasses of water half an hour before you eat at a restaurant.

Have An Early Appetiser

If you eat something about an hour before you head out you won't be ravenous when you arrive at the restaurant. Then, when ordering, always choose a starter of soup (minestrone, gazpacho, or anything chicken-broth-based) or a salad. Both options are low glycaemic (ie, digested slowly), so they won't spike blood sugar levels, which, can trigger food cravings.

Eat Somewhere Clean And Well-Lit

Stay out of dark steak houses. Researchers at the University of California at Irvine found that low lights increase binge eating. Dimmer lights make you less self-aware, which loosens your inhibitions, say the researchers.

Share Your Dessert

Go ahead and have something sweet for a treat, but share it with someone else, or, even better with two other people. Or, if no one wants to share, only eat half. If you can't do that, don't have dessert.

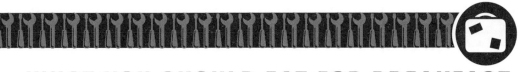

WHAT YOU SHOULD EAT FOR BREAKFAST

This is the easiest meal to manage healthily, because the food choices at a café or hotel breakfast buffet are so similar to what you eating at home. Give yourself enough time to eat a big breakfast. It'll start you on the right track for the day.

Avoid high-carbohydrate options such as pancakes, bagels, muffins and chips. Instead, start out with a fibre-packed bowl of porridge sweetened with a handful of raisins. Order a spinach and feta cheese omelette, one of the most nutritious choices on the menu (feta cheese has about a third less fat than cheddar). Avoid sausage and streaky bacon, go for back bacon and leave the rind behind. Toast? Wholemeal, of course.

WHAT YOU SHOULD EAT FOR LUNCH...

You can't go wrong with a salad for lunch if you control the dressings. But what if your party has decided on a burger or a sandwich? Here's how to get your order right.

...At The Sandwich Shop

First things first, choose wholemeal bread. Try to avoid anything with mayonnaise or processed meat – they're likely to be full of saturated fat. Go for grilled chicken with lots of salad: filling up on veggies can help you avoid getting hungry mid-afternoon. Skip the meal deals, or swap the crisps for fruit and fizzy drinks for water. Check nutrition labels on packaged sandwiches.

...At The Burger Joint

Forget about the fries, of course. You're better off ordering two regular burgers, dumping one bun, and making a double-decker. Hold the mayo. If you're eating at McDonald's or Burger King, choose the hamburger or a Whopper Jr instead of those fried fish fillet sandwiches. You'll save lots of calories and grams of fat.

EASY LIFESTYLE TWEAK

We go through a number of 90 minute cycles when we sleep. Setting your alarm for the end of one of these can help you wake up feeling refreshed and energised, giving you extra energy for your morning workout.

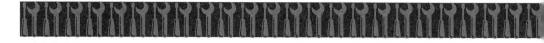

WHAT YOU SHOULD EAT FOR DINNER...

Here's where your habit of snacking healthily throughout the day can pay off. You'll find it easy to skip the deep-fried calamari appetiser and the béarnaise sauce on your steak. Having arrived at the restaurant without hunger pangs, you'll be a model of self-discipline. And you won't get butter drips on your shirt.

...At The Steak House

Grilled salmon is always an excellent choice, but if you want beef, go for sirloin or fillet. Both are less fatty than the rib eye. Ask for an extra vegetables instead of a chips. Or see if they can get you a baked sweet potato, which packs more fibre and vitamins than a spud. Start with a soup or salad to keep hunger at bay.

...At The Italian Restaurant

Start with antipasto cured meat for the protein. Bread sticks are much better than a basket of garlic bread, only a couple, mind. Share a pizza with someone else and order a side such as potato wedges or, even better, salad. This way you avoid eating a whole pizza to yourself which could easily push 2,000 calories.

...At The Seafood Restaurant

Easy to be good here, right? Yes, if you stay away from tartare sauce, which packs 10 grams of fat in a single tablespoon; fried crab cakes, fried shrimp, fried oysters (see a pattern?); creamy fish soup and, of course, chips. Eat instead grilled salmon, tuna, sea bass, almost anything grilled or steamed (but watch the butter). Tomato-based fish stews made with light broths are good starter choices, too. Always choose steamed vegetables and brown rice rather than fries.

...At the Indian

Check the menu for vegetable curries made with dal (stewed black lentils that are a terrific source of low-fat protein and fibre). Also look for dishes based on chickpeas, spinach, tomatoes, and

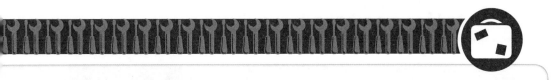

MAINTENANCE APPS

Keep your belly at bay forever

MEN'S HEALTH TRAINING PRO	EVERYDAY HEALTH	LOSE IT!	BODY HEALTH CALCULATOR
iPhone, free	iPhone, free	iPhone, free	iPhone, free
Sixteen iPhone-optimised 'how-to' videos along with instructions. Being shown what to do in a clear, step-by-step fashion, means you're exercising – and burning fat – more effectively. Yes, we know we're biased, but it's really very good.	A library of over 34,000 foods and their nutritional values, which will help you to keep track of what you're eating every single day. A recent UK study found blood sugar levels were more stable and metabolism higher when eating to a structured plan.	This calorie budgeter sets daily limits and calculates how many your level of activity is burning off. Great for long-term fitness plans. Research from Cornell University found the average diner underestimates how many calories they're eating by a whopping 38%.	Your BMI, body fat levels and metabolic rate all revealed in one app. It'll tell you where to work harder. Having precise data will allow you to set more specific goals and give you early warnings when you might be slipping off course. It's maintenance made easy.

mushrooms. Tomato-based options include jalfrezi, karahi or balti. They're much lower in calories than creamier dishes like masala, korma or makhani. Avoid lamb as it can be quite fatty.

...At The Chinese

Skip the prawn crackers, they contain one gram of fat each. Ask for brown rice instead of white rice to get more fibre. For your main course, choose stir fried vegetables and avoid anything called 'crispy' (deep fried) or anything in a gloopy sauce – they're packed full of fat. Use chopsticks instead of a fork. You'll eat more slowly and may end up eating less.

CASE STUDY

London-based IT worker **Michael Duong** turned fat burning into a personal challenge and left his old overweight self behind for good

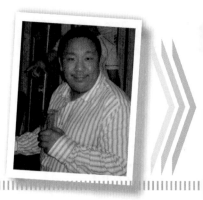

"I WAS THE FATTEST OF MY FRIENDS"

"Photographs at a party shocked me into action," says Michael. "I was by far the fattest among my friends. One of them had just lost 2st (13kg) and had become noticeably more attractive to women. I knew I had to change, too." Michael decided to use his social network as a way to ensure his fitness regime stayed on track. "One of my mates agreed to lose weight with me. We tracked our progress every two weeks in a table." Introducing a competitive element is an excellent tool for staying focused, so find a friend or

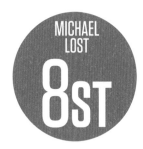

MICHAEL LOST

8ST

family member who'd also like to drop a few pounds and throw down the gauntlet.

As a way to ensure he never missed a workout, Michael introduced exercise into his everyday routine. "I now cycle to work and back – 30 miles a week in total. I also play five-a-side football every week." Keep burning fat without risking setbacks by basing 80% of your cardio around cycling. US studies show that unlike running, cycling on consecutive days does not raise your risk of overtraining or injury.

HIT BACK AT FAT

Michael also stopped his regime from becoming dull by introducing some high-adrenaline sport. "A mate who teaches kickboxing encouraged me to go to his classes. I was an easy target for the punches at first, which was the perfect inspiration to get back on my bike and get fitter. I never did weights, but I did try some bodyweight exercises like the pull-up hang. Once your chin is

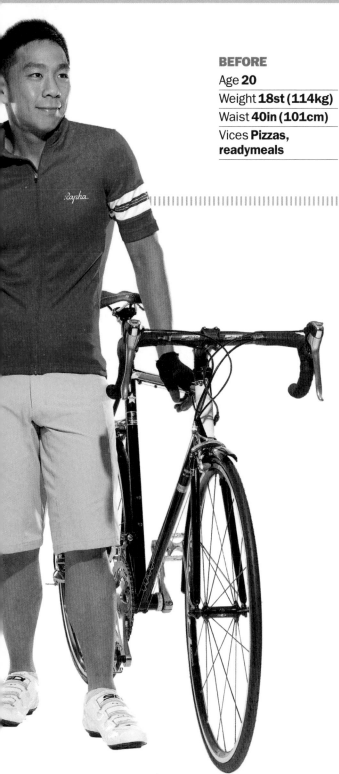

BEFORE	AFTER
Age **20**	Age **22**
Weight **18st (114kg)**	Weight **10st (63.5kg)**
Waist **40in (101cm)**	Waist **30in (75cm)**
Vices **Pizzas, readymeals**	Victories **Energy and confidence**

over the bar, you hold until you arms fail. Trust me, it's a lot harder than it sounds – especially when you weigh 18st."

EATING RIGHT

"I had no real appreciation of the nutrition. Carbs, proteins, they were all the same. Much of what I ate failed to fill me up, so I'd simply eat more." Now Michael has a better understanding of nutrition and often has low-carb days – a study at Manchester University showed cutting carbs just two days a week is a superior weight-loss method to cutting

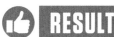 **RESULT**

"My life is unrecognisable. I have a genuine sense of energy and purpose," says Michael. "I feel a lot more confident and stronger – physically and mentally. Everybody tells me I look younger and I now have big goals within my reach, starting with a triathlon or half marathon."

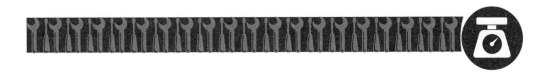

HOW TO STAY
LEAN
FOR LIFE

**NOW YOU'VE LOST YOUR BELLY HERE'S HOW
TO MAKE SURE IT NEVER COMES BACK**

CONGRATULATIONS. By now you've slimmed down and dramatically improved your fitness and your health. Go ahead and toast yourself with a ice cold lager or something else you've been craving. Do you really just want a Wagonwheel? Well, why not? You deserve it.

Now comes the tricky part: keeping the weight off for good. You'll gain it back in a hurry if you go back to your old ways. Fortunately, you've learned a thing or two about how your body responds to food, you've learned how to keep your metabolism running fast by eating small meals frequently throughout the day and you've made exercise a regular part of your lifestyle. And that lean muscle you've added to your frame helps fry calories even when you're sitting around on the sofa watching *MasterChef*.

OF COURSE, THERE'S ALWAYS THE DANGER of slipping back to belly central. A new job might mean tonnes of extra work. A new baby might keep you up all night. A twisted knee might keep you off the treadmill. All three of those things can happen very easily and they could even happen all at once. A ligament injury might keep you on the sofa, nursing your knee, munching your way through bags of double chocolate chip cookies. The excuses are easy, and it's really damaging to your fitness momentum and your motivation.

If you stop exercising, you can tend to get lazy in other parts of your life, especially your diet. When your life gets so badly disrupted by an injury, new arrival to the family or anything out of the ordinary it's easy to let your goals get out of reach, and join the ranks of the 80 percent of exercisers and dieters who fail to stick with their well-intended programmes.

The point is that setbacks are common and it's likely that you will struggle at times with finding the motivation and the time to maintain the gains (and losses) you've made with *The Fat Burner's Bible*. At times like these spending time online with the members of online health communities can really pay off. And you can always go back to where you started and recommit to the principles of the health and fitness programme set out in this book:

1. Spark your metabolism every morning with the 15-minute workout and a nutritious, protein-rich breakfast.

2. Eat small meals four to six times a day in order to stifle junk food cravings and bingeing.

3. Exercise with your bodyweight or barbells and do some cardiovascular interval training.

4. Avoid cakes, biscuits, and other processed foods, and focus on fibre-rich, nutrient-dense, whole grains, vegetables and fruits, plus have at least a little protein every time you eat. Limit carbs as much as possible after 6pm.

5. Limit your consumption of liquid calories, especially alcohol. (Congratulations, you can have beer and wine again! But keep consumption to three or four alcoholic beverages per week. Remember, carbs and alcohol in beer, wine and tequila slammers act like liquid fat, and that fat will hone right in to your belly.)

FAT BURNING SUPPS

THERE ARE NO MAGIC BULLETS, BUT THERE ARE SHORTCUTS...

BEST FOR
FIRST-TIME FAT BURNERS
Thermobol

A cocktail of several weight-loss heavy-hitters, such as L-tyrosine, caffeine and black pepper extract, it also contains guarana, which research in the *International Journal of Obesity* found can shift almost 3.4kg of fat in eight weeks. Maximuscle has also created a caffeine-free version.

£37, maximuscle.com

BEST FOR
EXTRA ENERGY
Biotest Hot-Rox Extreme

"It's a combination of journal-proven, metabolism-boosting ingredients, like yohimbine, Carbolin 19 and raspberry," says Brad Morris, a sports scientist and wrestling coach to the Australian rugby team Penrith Panthers. It'll give you extra energy so be just be careful when you take it – try it 30 minutes before training and you'll get an extra boost to power through your fat-blasting workouts.

£34, tmuscle.com

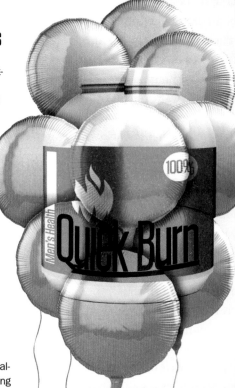

BEST FOR
IMPROVING WILLPOWER
Sci-MX Pyro-MX

This stops your weight issues at their source: your stomach. "Chromium and yerba mate suppress food cravings," says Morris. It also contains metabolism boosters, like white kidney bean extract. A study in the *Alternative Medicine Review* found this can shift ½lb (¼kg) a week.

£17, sci-mx.co.uk

BEST FOR
LAST RESORT
N-Cinerate

This product's USP is that it contains 15 fat-burning ingredients, which means there should be something in there that works for you. "They're all proven to reduce appetite, increase energy and cull fat," says Morris. This is perfect for the man who has tried everything – but still wants less.

£37, bodyactive-online.co.uk

BEST FOR
ANXIETY-FREE FAT LOSS
Venom Hyperdrive 3

This strips fat reserves without the jitters. It has high doses of weight-loss ingredients such as L-tyrosine, which a study in *Brain Research* found stops the body getting stressed when you cut calories. It also has 5-Hydroxytryptophan, to curb binge eating.

£36, bodyactive-online.co.uk

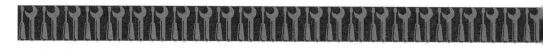

STICK WITH IT AND STAY LEAN FOR LIFE

Meanwhile, here are some motivational tips and tricks that we've collected from trainers, exercise physiologists, psychologists, and fellow dieters over the years that may help you to stick at it.

Use Visual Cues

Remember that 'before' photograph you took of yourself when you first picked up *The Fat Burner's Bible*? Hang it in a place where you'll see it every day. Now tape a photo of your new, thinner self next to the fat photo. There's visual motivation for you. Before and ever after. Share your success story with the world by posting your photos and story online. Nothing firms up a commitment like going public with it.

Weigh Yourself Every Day

It'll remind you of your goals and provide you with positive feedback. Remember what you learned in Chapter One: people who weighed themselves every day were 82 percent more likely to keep their weight off than people who didn't use scales, according to a recent study at the Weight Control and Diabetes Research Center in Providence, Rhode Island. For the most accurate readings, weigh yourself at the same time every day, since weight can fluctuate by several pounds at different times.

Eat A Pickle

When a craving for something salty and crunchy threatens your good intentions, reach for a pickle instead of the Pringles. Gherkins are low in calories and will cover both cravings.

Wake Up At 6:25

If you find you're skipping breakfast, wake up five minutes earlier. Five minutes is all you need to toast some bread or microwave some porridge. Remember that eating breakfast will help you eat less later in the day.

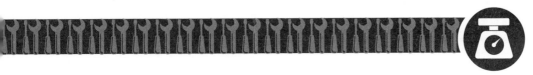

Put Money On Your Muscle

If you hired a personal trainer and cancelled a session without notice, you'd still have to pay the trainer. Treat yourself the same way. If you miss a workout, pay a spouse, friend or charity £10. Or pay yourself, say, £20 for every good workout. Stash the money in a fund, and reward yourself when you reach a weight-loss goal. Here's an idea: buy yourself some new clothes. You'll need them after losing all that weight.

If you don't think your disciplined enough for that, then make wager with a workout partner – first guy to wimp out pays up. In one study, people who bet they could stick to a workout programme for six months scored a 97 percent success rate (this compares very favourably with the average of 25 percent of people who have the necessary staying power).

Take That First Step

No matter how tired you are, exercise will make you feel better. Taking those first few steps after a tough day at work is difficult, but research shows that working out raises your energy levels and improves your mood.

Take A Day Off

Schedule a cheat day – Sunday, for example. It's a day where you rest and eat whatever you want. It will give you a psychological boost. If on Tuesday you really want an Aero, you know you have to wait until Sunday until you can have one. A cheat day is a technique used effectively for motivation even among professional models and athletes. Denying yourself food and drink that you love forever just isn't workable. Confining those treats to one day a week is. What's more, some studies suggest that eating stodgy carbohydrates (and, let's face it, that's what we usually crave) just occasionally can actually help to rev up your metabolism and make it run faster for days afterwards, aiding your fat-burning efforts in the long run. However, make sure you don't cheat more than a day a week.

EASY LIFESTYLE TWEAK

Buy some black-out blinds for your bedroom. Sleeping in the dark helps you have a more restful night's sleep, meaning you'll have more energy for fat-burning workouts the next day. Plus, if you are overtired you'll body will be flooded with hormones that make you extra hungry.

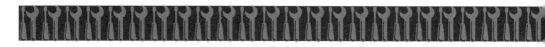

Schedule An Exercise Meeting

When work gets so busy that you have trouble fitting in a workout, schedule a running meeting with colleagues. Then you can multitask. This strategy is actually popular with the editors of *Men's Health* for brainstorming sessions. Some of our best ideas come out of lunchtime jogs round the parks near our London offices.

Crank Up The Techno

Reams of research show that if you work out to your favourite music, you'll work out longer and more intensely. In one study those who exercised to music lost 8lb (3.5kg) more than those who sweated in silence. What should you listen to? Whatever you like, but make it fast. The faster the tune you are listening to, the more vigorously you'll push yourself.

Chart Your Progress

Every time you complete a workout mark it off on a chart (you can use the one on the last page of this book). Or put workouts into your smart phone's calendar for reminder alerts – and don't forget to check back to get the satisfaction of seeing how many workouts you've completed. Researchers who tested this system found that exercisers who tracked their workouts were more successful at sticking with their plans than those who didn't. There is also space to record your weight. But probably more important is your waist measurement. This is the best instant indication of how much fat you have lost. What's more, seeing your belly disappear, centimetre by centimetre will encourage you to stick with the programme.

But it's not just about satisfaction. There's a practical element to recording your workouts, too. For this it pays buy a notebook or diary and record the reps you do and weights you use, if any, for each exercise. Do it as you work out. Then, when you come to your next workout you can quickly flip back and see what you achieved last time. You should always be aiming to do a little bit more with each workout. If you don't constantly give your body new challenges your weight loss and muscle building will stall.

GYM TIP

Try jogging through water, whether it's at your local pool, or in the sea. It will burn twice the calories of running on land, so you can finish your workout in half the time.

GOOD LUCK AND THE BEST OF HEALTH!

The biggest lesson to learn through any diet and exercise programme is that the effort doesn't end once you reach your goal. There's no finish line. It's a new lifestyle. Every day for the rest of your life, you will make better food choices and find ways to be active. It will all come naturally because it will make you feel great.

We hope that you have found the tools, techniques, and inspiring testimonials in this book useful for reaching your weight-loss goals. As mentioned in Chapter One, and you'll know from experience, there are no magic bullets – no pills, potions, fad denial diets or pieces of revolutionary workout equipment that will do the work for you. The ultimate secret to achieving a healthy weight and fit body is your commitment to yourself. You are the X factor for success. If you want to feel better, look fitter, sidestep the diseases of ageing and live longer, you need to make your fitness a priority in your busy life. *The Fat Burner's Bible* can help. The real world weight-loss strategies used by the men in this book attack the fat that matters most, the dangerous belly fat that threatens your long-term health.

Our programme is designed to build a foundation of habits that become part of who you are. But everyone needs a refresher now and then, so we hope that you will refer back to this book when you need a tip, want to check an exercise technique, or just need some inspiration when life's jam doughnuts beckon you away from eating right. For added support get onto the *Men's Health* website where you can meet other readers who are eager to burn fat or maintain the weight loss they've already achieved. Just log onto the weight loss forum at **menshealth.co.uk/fatburnerforum** You can swap workout tips and recipes and get advice on maintaining motivation and, who knows? You may get just the boost you need to power you towards achieving even greater success – like Fat Burner of the Month Dave Leather, who became a finalist in the *Men's Health* Cover Model Competition. Whatever happens, the camaraderie of the weight-loss community will make your own challenge easier, more fun and very rewarding.

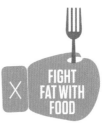

FIGHT FAT WITH FOOD

Go slow and steady, don't wolf down your food. A study at the University of Rhode Island, USA, found slow eaters ate about 67 fewer calories per meal.

CASE STUDY

Anthony Lawton, a musician from Doncaster, skewered his lager and kebab lifestyle for a healthier regime that torched blubber

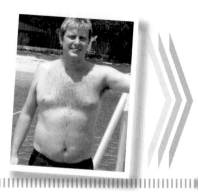

"FAT WAS THREATENING MY JOB"

Anthony's lifestyle left him feeling low. Working as a touring musician he would hit the booze after gigs: "I'd finished my show late at night and follow it with five pints and a kebab. I'd have a fry-up breakfast in the morning and eat burgers and chips for meals".

Not only did Anthony's lifestyle affect his weight, it also began to affect his work and his asthma: "I was fat, which made my asthma worse and affected my saxophone playing. It was threatening my livelihood as well as my health".

Anthony was determined to get into shape and transform his life. His love of competition helped him get into an exercise routine that fitted around his work. "Weekly five-a-side sessions when not touring re-ignited my love of cardio. I now go to the gym at 7am when the machines are free and then do swimming intervals".

CAVEMAN FOOD

Not only did he change his exercise routine, but his diet as well. Before his weight loss, Anthony was eating a fry-up for breakfast, a carb-filled lunch and a burger and chips for dinner. Now, his new regime keeps him off the junk and feeling great. "I follow the Paleolithic 'caveman' diet eating six meals a day with a 50/30/20 : protein/fat/carb split. Mackerel or chicken for lunch and a large carb intake after training".

Anthony noticed an improvement not only in his appearance, but also in his mind set. He now has more energy, greater confidence and his saxophone technique is better than ever before.

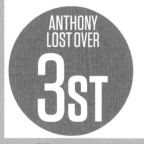

ANTHONY LOST OVER

3ST

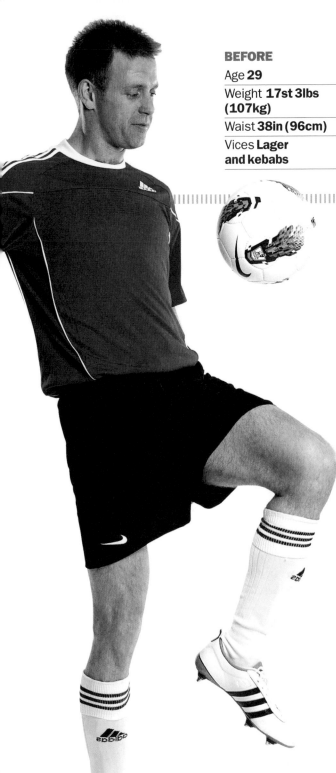

BEFORE	AFTER
Age **29**	Age **30**
Weight **17st 3lbs** **(107kg)**	Weight **13st 11lbs** **(87kg)**
Waist **38in (96cm)**	Waist **32in (81cm)**
Vices **Lager** **and kebabs**	Victories **More** **energy**

A FRESH START

Now Anthony is gearing up for the future: "I have really enjoyed this journey and I know it isn't over as I still have goals and targets I want to achieve. I would one day love to compete on a triathalon or maybe swim a long distance for charity".

But even that won't be the end for Anthony. "I still read up in *Mens Health*," he says. "I love the tips I pick up on training and nutrition. I know this is my way of life now, and whilst its a long long road I am loving the ride and will be on it for the duration".

👍 RESULT

Trimming down helped Anthony fight his asthma and gain energy and confidence. "Losing a stone in the first couple of months made me psychologically stronger and more productive as a person. Now I am fitter and stronger than I've ever been in my life! I am totally focused on achieving my goals, no matter how difficult they seem."

INDEX

S

Salad 148, 150-151, 152

Salad dressing 40

Salmon 174

Sardines 174

Saturated fat 66-68

Sausages 40

Scales 119

Sea-bass 154

Seeds 174

Sex 33

Shopping 74-75

Shoulder press 123

Shoulder press-up 101

Side-to-side hops 81

Side-to-side shuffle 210

Simon Lim 188-189

Single-arm row 124

Single-leg hip extension 108

Six-Pack 30, 193-199

Skipping 216

Snacks 54, 58, 158-159

Soup 40

Spider-man press-up 108

Split Squat 106

Sprinter's step drill 207

Steak 153, 236

Step-up 99, 101, 206

Stretching 112-113

Sucrose 59

Sugar 38-42

Superman 199

Supplements 59-60, 243

Swimming 19, 110

Swiss ball 96-101

Swiss ball crunch 127

Swiss ball leg curl 107

Swiss ball press 126

Swiss ball rotation 107

T

T-pushup 206

Tea 174

Testosterone 33

Tim Ursell 160-161

Tomatoes 175

Trans fats 66-67

Trunk twist 196

Tuna 175

Turkey burgers 146

Turkey chilli 157

Two-minute drill 80-83

U

Upper-body shuttle 208

V

Vitamins 65

W

Walking lunge 126-127

Walking press-up 105

Water 44, 47

Watermelon 175

Weighted crunch 198

Weights 120-130, 217

Wholemeal 59, 167, 235

Y

Yoghurt 40, 139, 175

Z

Zinc 65

IMAGE CREDITS

All workouts:© Rodale
All case studies: Studio 33 (except p24 - David Venni)
All illustrations: Paul Aarons (unless credited below)

p29: I hate pies: Dan Matthews
p31: Portion sizes - Dan Matthews, food stylist;
    Nicholas Ghirlando
p32: Supplement balti - Jobe Lawrenson
p35: Scales - Sam Armstrong
p36: Trainers - Studio 33
p39: Chocolate runner - Sam Armstrong
p41: Eggs - David Newton
p42: Guinness ice-cream - Sam Armstrong
p45: Bar Chart - Hearst
p47 : Ice Trophy - Peter Crowther Associates
p60: Hit or Myth - Jason Pickersgill at acutegraphics.co.uk
p69: Fish of fish - Johanna Parkin; food stylist Maud Eden
p75-77: Food - Studio 33, Maria Jefferis, William Shaw,
        Michael Jennison, Sliced banana, Jon Whitaker,
        Clive Streeter
p97: Swiss ball - Studio 21
p138: Bacon and Egg Muffin - Natmags
p139: Quick Thick Yoghurt - David Munns
p140: Protein-power Porridge - Joy Skipper
p142: Country Omelette - Jon Whitaker
p143: Hot Breakfast Burrito - Jon Whitaker
p144: Mediterranean Wrap - RGB Digital
p145: Prawn and Pasta Salad - Gareth Morgans
p146: Turkey Burgers - Kate Whitaker
p148: Greek Salad - Studio 33
p150-151: Spinach Salad - Jon Whitaker
p152: Turkey-Avocado Salad - Jon Whitaker
p153: Super Sirloin Steak - William Shaw
p154: Sea Bass - David Munns
p156: Stuffed Chicken - Steve Baxter
p157: Turkey Chilli - Ian Garlick
p165: Almonds - Webster Shooter
    Apples - Olle Svensson
    Asparagus - William Shaw
    Avocado - Tony Briscoe
p166: Bananas - Studio 33
    Beans - Studio 33
    Beef - Studio 33
    Beetroot - Studio 33

p167: Blueberries - RW
    Bread - Wiliam Shaw
    Chillies - Claire Richardson
p168: Chocolate - Lisa Gee for Studio 33
    Edamame - Joyosity
p169: Hummus - Studio 21
    Kiwis - Sandra Lane
p170: Nuts - Studio 21
    Oats - Studio 33
    Olive oil - Cosmo Hair UK
p171: Onions - Lizzie Orme
    Papayas - Studio 33
p172: Pears - Jon Whitaker
    Peppers - Mike McClafferty
    Pork chops - Ian Garlick
p173: Quinoa - Charlotte Tolhurst
    Rice - Tony Briscoe
    Rocket - flickr user Tim Lewis
p174: Salmon - Ian Garlick
    Sardines - Jon Whitaker
    Seeds - Brian Jackson
    Tea - David Martyn Hunt
p175: Tomatoes - Studio 33
    Yoghurt - Studio 33
    Watermelon - Rob White
p176: Jacket potato with fork - Getty
p182: Muesli - Jon Whitaker
    Camembert - Sam Stowell
    Spinach - Studio 33
p183 : Energy Drinks - Max Oppenheim
    Cauliflower - William Shaw
p184: Popcorn - Johanna Parkin
    Sunglasses - Lisa Gee for Studio 33
p185: Spring onions - Iain Bagwell
p186: Lentils - Studio 33
    Protein powder - Studio 33
p187: Smoothie - Gareth Morgans
    Black pepper - Studio 33
p195: Six-Pack - Studio 33
p229: Suitcase - Coneyl Jay
p232-233: Buffet - Mitch Mandel and Thomas
        MacDonald/Rodale Images
p243: Balloon supplements -
    Spooky Pooka @ Debut Art

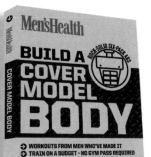
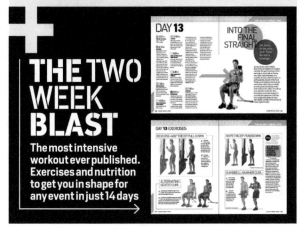

Pick the best food, wherever you are

You can eat burgers AND lose pounds with this amazing new nutrition guide from the editors of **Men'sHealth**

EAT THIS NOT THAT!

Big Mac
490 Calories
24g fat

SAVE more than 240 calories & nearly 20g of fat

Whopper with cheese
734 Calories
43g fat

- ☑ Thousands of surprising food swaps!
- ☑ The best foods to eat at your favourite restaurants
- ☑ Your healthiest ever supermarket shopping list
- ☑ Delicious recipes guaranteed to beat the bulge

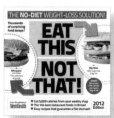

The quick way to supercharge your fat-burning

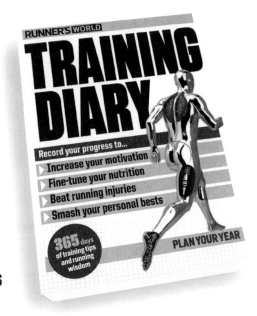

- ☑ **Record every run you make**
- ☑ **Improve race times**
- ☑ **Easy-to-use, any-year format**
- ☑ **52 weeks of advice from the pros**
- ☑ **The latest training science**

ORDER YOUR COPY NOW

HEARSTSUBS.CO.UK/RW/BM07
OR CALL 0844 848 1601 AND QUOTE BM07

£9.99
FREE P&P*
*UK orders only. Please allow 21 days for delivery

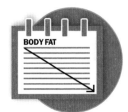

BODY FAT

PROGRESS LOG

Keeping track of your weight loss is great motivation. When you complete a workout, write in the space provided **C** = Cardio, **B100** = Bodyweight 100, **B200** = Bodyweight 200, **SS** = Supersets, **W** = Weights Workout

	WEEK ONE	WEEK TWO	WEEK THREE	WEEK FOUR
Weight				
Waist				
Monday				
Tuesday				
Wednesday				
Thursday				
Friday				
Saturday				
Sunday				

	WEEK FIVE	WEEK SIX	WEEK SEVEN	WEEK EIGHT
Weight				
Waist				
Monday				
Tuesday				
Wednesday				
Thursday				
Friday				
Saturday				
Sunday				

	WEEK NINE	WEEK TEN	WEEK ELEVEN	WEEK TWELVE
Weight				
Waist				
Monday				
Tuesday				
Wednesday				
Thursday				
Friday				
Saturday				
Sunday				